The Chaplain's Conflict

Number 137: Williams-Ford
Texas A&M University Military History Series

The Chaplain's Conflict

Good and Evil in a War Hospital, 1943–1945

Tennant McWilliams

Texas A&M University Press
College Station

First edition

This paper meets the requirements of ANSI/NISO Z39.48-1992 (Permanence of Paper).
Binding materials have been chosen for durability.

Library of Congress Cataloging-in-Publication Data

McWilliams, Tennant S., 1943–
The chaplain's conflict : good and evil in a war hospital, 1943–1945 / Tennant McWilliams.—1st ed.
p. cm.
The author based the book on Rev. Kennedy's letters, war diaries, and post-war magazine articles, as well as a personal yearlong trip retracing Kennedy's war locales, including conducting interviews with local citizens about their war remembrances.
Includes bibliographical references and index.
ISBN-13: 978-1-60344-470-5 (cloth : alk. paper)
ISBN-10: 1-60344-470-X (cloth : alk. paper)
ISBN-13: 978-1-60344-689-1 (e-book)
ISBN-10: 1-60344-689-3 (e-book)
1. Kennedy, Renwick C., 1900?–1985. 2. United States. Army. Evacuation Hospital, 102nd. 3. World War, 1939–1945—Chaplains—United States. 4. United States. Army—Chaplains. 5. Military chaplains—United States. 6. Military chaplains—Presbyterian Church. 7. World War, 1939–1945—Personal narratives, American. 8. World War, 1939–1945—Campaigns—Western Front. 9. World War, 1939–1945—Regimental histories—United States. I. Title.
D810.C36U66 2012
940.54'78092—dc23

2011034421

Susan joins me in dedicating this book to Marc and Béatrice Ferri
of Paris and Pennedepie.

Contents

Acknowledgments

For their friendship and long-time support of this book, I am grateful to Mary Conway Kennedy Dickinson, of Atmore, Alabama, and Margaret Kennedy Ausley, of Nokesville, Virginia. That they are so devoted to their father's memory, while so fervently analytical about him, is a lesson I am still digesting. I suspect genetics.

Far across the Atlantic others have provided significant research assistance alongside heartfelt international friendship: Louis Forget, mayor of Jullouville, France; Jean-Christophe and Régine Coppée of Ochamps, Belgium; Christine Bouchon of Paris and Bazenville, France; Graham and Isabelle Wilson of Barneville-la-Bertran, France; Sylvie Louboutin-Croc of Ploudaniel, France; Marie Louise Lévi-Ménard of Bréville-sur-Mer, France; and certainly Marc and Béatrice Ferri of Paris and Pennedepie, France, to whom this book is dedicated. Each day for more than a year with trust and extraordinary kindness Marc and Béatrice welcomed two—heretofore unknown—Americans into the warmth and history of their family's Pennedepie château, Val Fontaine.

An interdisciplinary scholarly community gave vital assistance. As detailed in the commentary on sources, staffs of wide-ranging libraries and archives as always proved enthusiastic. But special thanks indeed go to John Brinsfield and Marsha McManus of the US Army Chaplaincy Center Library at Fort Jackson, South Carolina; Matthew Tinker of the Southport (England) Public Library; Jerry W. Stephens, Brooke Becker, Eddie Luster, Patty Pilkerton, and Kelly Schiff of the Mervyn H. Sterne Library of the University of Alabama at Birmingham (UAB); and to everyone of those folks—many of whom are Vietnam veterans—at the Military Archives Division of the National Archives in College Park, Maryland. Those who helped me understand medical education, medical personnel, and medical issues of wartime include Clifton Meador of the Vanderbilt University School of Medicine; two World War II veterans—Wayne

Finley of the University of Alabama at Birmingham School of Medicine and Zachary Friedenberg of the University of Pennsylvania School of Medicine; Judith Bellafaire of the US Army Center for Military History in Washington, DC; and, especially for his cogent comments on pathology labs and "bug juice," Jay McDonald, also of the University of Alabama at Birmingham School of Medicine. In addition, UAB history colleagues James F. Tent and Robert Jefferson guided me at crucial junctures (Jim on a variety of military-history matters, Robert on the amazing story of Vasco Hale—a story still unfolding). Also, UAB medical sociologist and retired US Army general William C. Cockerham—a Vietnam veteran—counseled me on wide-ranging issues of army life. Likewise, Fred Fey of the Ettelbruck Agricultural College aided significantly on the 102nd Evacuation Hospital's movements immediately preceding the Battle of Bastogne, and Edward Russell, a Vietnam veteran with potent scholarly knowledge of World War II, advised me on unit and troop movements. Scott Schoner of the US Army Medical Museum at Fort Sam Houston in San Antonio helped greatly on the history of evacuation hospitals. Steve Padgett-Vasquez applied his formidable talents with satellite imaging to cartographic displays. Leo Ticheli of Ticheli Productions of Birmingham stole time away from making advertisements for General Motors to give magical (almost scary) renaissance to damaged wartime photographs. Two other Birmingham colleagues counseled on difficult matters of French-English translation: William C. Carter, University Distinguished Professor Emeritus at the University of Alabama at Birmingham (UAB), and Magalie Minaud, of the faculty of Indian Springs School. And the research assistance provided by Alexander Cohn, Adam Pinson, and John Boone was superb.

There also were crucial conversations. Long talks on the front porch at Oak Hill, Alabama, with Robert and Juliette Harper Bullock continue to help me probe the complicated terrains of Ren Kennedy's Christianity and social philosophy—which I am exploring more fully in a biography of him. Haas Strother of Camden, Alabama, assisted in much the same way. Too, in her vast knowledge of Wilcox County, Betty Gaines Kennedy—no relation to Ren Kennedy—helped me understand Kennedy's personality in the context of wartime Camden. Often with my two brothers, Richebourg and Burk, I got this instruction late on Saturday nights after the crowd was dwindling down at her venerable white-columned salon, the Gaines Ridge Supper Club. Similarly, Jean Touzé, of Angomesnil, France, on two occasions (with the *crucial* translation of Louis Forget) gave detailed accounts and a map of the 102nd Evacuation Hospital operations in and around Saint-Pair-sur-Mer, riveting detail matched only by other Saint-Pair accounts from Marie-Thérèse Provost Desroches, Roland Dulins Duprey, Claudie LeMaître, Yvette Bindel Gilbert, and Dominique Bindel Lucas, as well as Ploudaniel accounts by the late Georges Talec and by Daniel Berthou. No less engaging was Russell Summerlin of Delta, Alabama, without whom I would never have happened upon the full pathos of Kennedy's connection to the Lumpkin family. Finally, Edith Brawley, archivist of Erskine College, was an amazing help with records of the ARP church.

Virtually every university press in America has been hit hard by the recession, including Texas A&M University Press. Still, in helping birth *The Chaplain's Conflict,* the verve and vision of this press has been extraordinary. It's hard for an author to imagine more professional and encouraging people to work with than Mary Lenn Dixon, Thom Lemmons, and Carol Hoke.

Finally, it was Howell Raines who confided, "Just tell the tale—not only what happened to Ren but to you." I've tried to do that. Whatever the strengths of this story, however, it should be abundantly clear that Susan, with her love of the French language and well-honed intuition for understanding human predicaments, was key to it all—much to our mutual and enduring joy. As for dissenting opinions the book may invoke, especially in that it does not uniformly comport with Tom Brokaw's widely read and appropriately acclaimed *The Greatest Generation,* I can only say that Ren Kennedy compulsively tried to tell the truth about what he experienced in World War II, and I, compulsively, tried to tell the truth about what Ren told.

The Chaplain's Conflict

Overture

Goodbye, Farewell, Amen

Between 1972 and 1983 the heralded television series *M*A*S*H* brought America's public face to face with one of the most engaging elements of citizen soldiery: life inside an evacuation hospital. Even today reruns depicting the fictional 4077th evac enjoy a virtual cult following. A website permits international debate on the "true intent" of key monologues, and *M*A*S*H* theme parties punctuate wide-ranging social life. Regardless of his striking talents as actor, director, and producer, Alan Alda forever remains Benjamin Franklin ("Hawkeye") Pierce.

On the night of February 18, 1983, I was among those millions who watched the final *M*A*S*H* episode—"Goodbye, Farewell, and Amen." As a young historian I was self-consciously enthralled at being "present" at "the end." I had gone to Washington, DC, to a conference. With three old friends I went down to Georgetown to a pub with a small television set back in a smoky nook. After "the end" we ruminated about the way *M*A*S*H* people used brilliant humor to hook an audience into lucid lectures on changing values in American life, as if outlining James H. Whittebols's superb *Watching M*A*S*H, Watching America* (1998). But we also talked about the 4077th's evac story as a metaphor for war much as William Faulkner used a "postage stamp" of a Mississippi county to explore "universals." For through *M*A*S*H* many of the essential ingredients of war got center stage—if less so actual combat, still war's comedy and tragedy, courage and cowardliness, humility and hubris, and even deeper its life, death, necessity, and futility. Heavy thoughts that night in Georgetown.

A quarter of a century later I am thinking differently. Though still mesmerized by *M*A*S*H* reruns, I am thinking that while this noted *fictional* evac lives on, the *historical* evac of World War II, Korea, and Vietnam—whether a metaphor or simply a profound vehicle for saving lives—is dead. Indeed, it's past time we said goodbye, farewell, and amen and for the most part "job well done" to one of the most significant things ever adopted by the US Army. In the 1970s the army by necessity began focusing more on asymmetrical or guerilla warfare as opposed to conventional warfare with fighting on one side of a line and nonfighting on the other. In turn, as found in recent Middle East fighting, the evacuation hospital gave way to the "buddy aid" and "self-aid" strategies of *every* soldier—not just a member of the Army Special Forces—trained and equipped as a sophisticated emergency medical technician and helicopters triaging wounded back to a combat support hospital well removed from the fighting. Certainly "evacuation" remains a key ingredient of army medicine. However, it would take a return to old-style warfare to justify the rebirth of the historic evac, and just a glance at modern war technologies, not to mention contemporary geopolitics, makes this prospect unlikely.

History's farewell salute to the noble evac evokes complex memories. From army documents, several key books on US military medicine, and memoirs of doctors and nurses we recall that the US Army urged gearing up evacuation hospitals, or evacs, in the earliest stages of World War II. As the fighting commenced in North Africa, however, the evacs did not just appear. They had long been evolving out of the "flying hospitals" of Napoleon Bonaparte's chief of military surgery, Dominique Jean Larrey, then from Jonathan Letterman's lifesaving strategies of the American Civil War, and further refinements by both American and French doctors in World War I. In that context, the army's chief surgeon overseeing medicine in the North Africa, Mediterranean and European theaters, Maj. Gen. Paul R. Hawley, carefully analyzed lifesaving in North Africa campaigns. Then, in early 1943 he further refined the "chain of evacuation" concept into that famous sequence of military health care: from the field hospital to the evacuation hospital and on to station and general hospital, with the evac treating soldiers who might be returned to the front while evacuating on up the chain the more seriously wounded. As World War II unfolded, the army ultimately mounted some 107 of these units. Six emerged out of hospital and medical-school leaders imbued with "duty" approaching Major General Hawley and his colleagues: "We want to staff an evacuation hospital." From Margaret Bourke-White's photos in *Life* magazine in 1943, two books, and the amazing archival development of the University of North Carolina–Charlotte, none of these remains more prominent than the 38th Evacuation Hospital out of Charlotte, North Carolina. The other 101, however, emerged from top to bottom with the army's own strategic planning.

The army designed evacs to handle a maximum of either 400 or 600 patients. Sometimes functioning out of liberated brick facilities—schools, hotels, châteaux—more often they operated out of thirty to sixty tents. Tent life had the advantage of moving around patients all on one level—the ground. Usually lacking elevators, brick facilities had resultant problems of stairwells but were warmer and drier. Always at least semimobile, they used trucks, truck-style ambulances, and Jeeps and for long runs the railroads to stay optimally some eight miles back from actual fighting. They were staffed by male doctors—the smaller evacs with thirty, the larger ones up to fifty—mainly surgeons but also general-medicine physicians, as well as one or two anesthesiologists, optometrists, radiologists, and psychiatrists, and three to five dentists. They also had thirty-five to fifty female nurses all with nursing diplomas but most without baccalaureate degrees. Too, they included ten to fifteen college-educated officers to manage finances, supplies, engineering, chaplaincy, and the unit's other nonmedical affairs, as well as between 250 and 400 enlisted men, most with high-school educations to move the unit from place to place as war developments dictated. As detailed in a classic army manual, *Medical Field Manual: Mobile Units of the Medical Department* (1942), these truly were moving hospitals with wards for shock, surgery, post-op, usually a pharmacy, and even a morgue with pathology capabilities. If the *Manual* prescribed an ideal configuration for such medical camps, its priority goals of saving lives and winning a war urged that "seldom will the ideal arrangement be possible, nor will the various factors in any two situations be identical." By the time of the Korean conflict, the army had fine-tuned these operations and replaced the evac designation with "MASH"—mobile army surgical hospital.

A farewell salute to the evac also conjures up wide-ranging commentary. Start with *M*A*S*H.* Though essentially fiction set in Korea (increasingly influenced by cynicism over Vietnam), the show evolved out of a novel reflecting select interviews with former army surgeons plus some of the lead actors' own military experiences. It then skillfully probed the tensions of daily life in evacs as citizen-soldiers encountered moral dilemmas about war and other visceral issues with "establishment" types of both the career army and civilian life. In doing this, however, *M*A*S*H* never drew from the full extent of gore, trauma, and tragedy so integral to life in most evacs. Even if the film and television standards of that day had permitted such unvarnished realism about the most evil side of war—horrific death, for example, as later delivered in the opening scenes of *Saving Private Ryan*—the striking humor that *M*A*S*H* makers used to capture their audience would have seemed untenable alongside such disturbing truth.

In this vein recent military-history scholarship, while rarely read by the general public, offers extraordinary insight into active-duty soldiers, as well as veterans, and confronts the most visceral psychosocial implications of war. The general reading public, however, energized by *M*A*S*H* reruns, gets its revered "evac story" from wide-ranging memoirs of evac-based doctors and nurses, and these, in general, seem benignly one sided. They are strong on the civic duty, courage, talent, endurance, and humor so prominent in evac experiences. They are lacking in cases that involved darker developments: extreme gore and graphic death, serious drug and alcohol abuse, suicide, sexual violence, friendly-fire casualties, and other, just moronic deaths of comrades, as well as gross professional pettiness and discrimination on matters of gender, sexual orientation, and race. A veteran's understandable reluctance to relive such horrible experiences helps explain some of these holes in reality. So might the fact that most health-care providers were indoctrinated in the authority and goodness of their endeavors—much like some historians?—creating intense loyalties uncomfortable with public testimony about unsavory behavior within the profession. Long-standing military standards of protecting the sanctity of the command probably intensify this general lack of balance. So do historic army protocols (at times violated) banning war-zone diaries and letters of strategic substance. Perhaps even the recent syndrome of malpractice litigation indirectly enshrouds evac recollections. In short, if published memoirs as a genre are true and the *M*A*S*H* series brilliantly insightful, virtually all those telling the evac story to the public still have left out some fundamental stuff—with the evac's farewell left lacking.

That is, until now. As it turns out, yet another evac soldier now is poised to testify. His evac portrait is fuller than others because it is based on the firsthand, unfiltered private observations of someone outside the health-care professions and certainly one unworried about traditional strictures on the media. It is fuller because it derives from a beautifully educated character, in his midforties more mature than virtually everyone in his unit, and one who before going to war spent some sixteen years counseling a wide range of people on life and death and good and evil. It is fuller because he was a compulsive chronicler of the minute details of daily life. His name was Renwick C. Kennedy. Close friends called him

Ren. With Ren's salute added to the farewell the story goes deeply and fairly into the most fundamental issues of war.

Before I give you this true evac story, however, I need to tell you how I came by it—for that is part of its truth. Here's the brief version.

In September 1961, just before starting college, I drove from Birmingham down to Oak Hill, a tiny place in Wilcox County, Alabama, to talk with my Uncle Bill and Aunt Joyce about bringing some friends to hunt in the late fall. That afternoon as I headed up the road to the house Uncle Bill was on the front porch, slowly moving back and forth in one of those dark green rockers. So was Renwick C. Kennedy—minister at the Associate Reformed Presbyterian church down the road. I urged Mr. Kennedy to keep his seat, which he didn't do. He shook my hand and chatted with me as if we had talked many times before. Even though he and my father were close friends, however, I really don't think we had. I recall his stature that day as just under six feet. I also remember his accent—a rounded blend of Old South and Ivy League—as well as his softly syncopated pauses even in midsentence to choose just the right adjective. At any rate, to let them complete whatever was on their minds, I went on back through the house to the kitchen to visit with Aunt Joyce. Some ten minutes passed. I heard Mr. Kennedy's car start, and shortly Uncle Bill joined us at the kitchen table.

When I casually asked how Mr. Kennedy was doing, Uncle Bill just said, "Still the smartest man I've ever known." Perhaps because I had college on my mind I said something like, "You're a graduate of Columbia University, and he's the smartest man you ever met?" Just staring at me he repeated, "Still the smartest man I've ever known." A longtime educator always hungry for a "teaching moment," he then went to his study and returned with a late 1940s' issue of *Time* magazine. "Here, look at this." Knowing the interrogation ahead, I read it carefully—how the editors of *Time* had come across a recent article in *Christian Century* by this Alabama preacher named Kennedy and how Kennedy's scathing criticism of certain army behaviors in World War II fitted into a slowly bubbling-up realism about "the war." At that time Vietnam was below the public's radar. Hence, World War II as "a good war"—what an odd thing to say about any war, necessary or not—had not fully jelled. However, we still talked for hours as Uncle Bill, a proud veteran of the American Expeditionary Force in World War I, recalled Ren in December of 1945 sitting in that same dark green rocker ("Ren's rocker—that uncomfortable, double-seated one") out front quietly trying to sort out his recent life as a chaplain in the US Army's 102nd Evacuation Hospital—from Normandy to the Battle of the Bulge and on to the liberation of Germany.

Time passed. Remember, this is the short version. Ultimately, I found that Ren Kennedy had done far more than write a high-profile article about World War II, one that the great Princeton historian Eric Goldman focused upon in his 1956 classic, *The Crucial Decade—and After.* When Kennedy died in 1985, he left me his papers. From interviews with him I knew the collection existed in boxes scattered all over his house in Camden, Alabama, thirteen miles north of our place at Oak Hill. But what I found was staggering—the gigantic product of an addicted chronicler. Spanning the years from 1927 to 1983 were five thousand letters (to and from), plus sermons and diaries with detailed recordings on how his world unfolded each day: his reactions to the first two chapters of William Faulkner's *Absalom, Absalom!;* his lingering at our dining room table at Oak Hill to discuss with Uncle Bill the new book *Savage Symphony,* in which Eva Lips recounted the tragedy of an anthropologist's struggling to tell the truth under Nazism; what several congregation members thought of his Easter sermon "this morning"; the weather—"23 degrees at 1:00 AM, cloudy but no ice"; oh, the weather—all together some eighteen hundred recordings over fifty-six years, always followed by bed around 2:00 AM. When packed up for moving, the diaries alone filled six cardboard whiskey boxes. More to the point, through his letters and diaries this scholarly preacher had recorded in striking realism what he had experienced with the 102nd Evac. By comparison, this made the unit's official records in the National Archives at best a skeletal, if still crucial, account.

Because Ren was a preacher, I need to make something clear. He was a moralist, as well as a realist. In the year before he joined the army he laid out his moralism about war in a guest sermon at Oak Hill. Different pieces of this sermon he then used throughout the war. Titling the sermon "The Christian and the War," he explained that "in modern war you kill indiscriminately men, women, and children. . . . You machine-gun the fleeing populace. To war nothing whatsoever is sacred and anything at all may be violated. . . . Jesus said killing was a sin [and] war is the supreme collective sin of the human race." However, after arguing that violent fascism also was a sin and that Hitler could be the anti-Christ, he said he personally gave strong support to Americans who were fighting in the war. "The State is waging the war, not the church, and I am a citizen of the State. The State

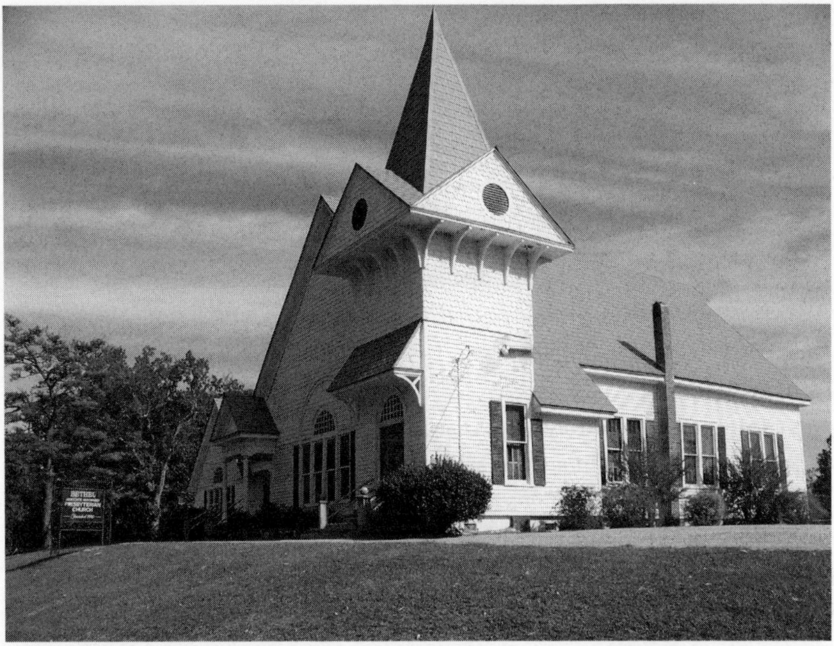

Contemporary view of Bethel Associate Reformed Presbyterian Church in Oak Hill, Alabama, where RCK first gave his "Christian and the War" sermon, April 19, 1942. Photo by Susan McWilliams.

guarantees to the church the right to practice religion [and] this guarantee carries with it certain responsibilities to the State." Further, if "American entry into the war violates Christianity, the alternative promises to violate it still more [and] I choose between the two evils and support the war."

Ren saw the "means" versus the "ends" of war through similar moralism. In the same sermon at Oak Hill he emphasized that people fighting a war for civilized behavior must not let that endeavor make them as uncivilized and insensitive as the cause they sought to defeat. In fact, he viewed the otherwise "good" outcome of World War I—the necessary defeat of Germany—fully offset by the "evil" means by which the Treaty of Versailles greedily gave England and France virtually all of Germany's economic assets, then created a weak League of Nations unable to deal with the resultant "mess": "We and the rest of the nations [Britain, France] have made the world patterned after the selfish will of man, clogged with evils—social, economic, political, racial, religious. . . . [World War II] is not God's will [but] it is His Judgment coming inexorably upon men in consequent of their violation of His spiritual laws." The man could preach. Still, Ren was anything *but* a prudish Victorian fitting the (unjustified) stereotype of the army chaplain. He was a modern Christian. For him there was no contradiction between science and religion and, as I earlier mentioned about his approach to the war, no paralysis about acting "sinful" if that helped address a greater problem. Rarely did he seek segregation from the things that have always happened in war and always will. An intellectual as much as a preacher, he was at once fascinated with war and perplexed by its implications for good and evil not just for the world abstractly but also for himself concretely.

The truth is that he was even more than fascinated. He was *compulsively* fascinated. So, what about those army protocols about a soldier on the front writing down details that, if captured by the enemy, could prove more than costly? It's hard to say whether his Princeton-educated intellect aided or abetted him. Perhaps both—to the good of history. Suffice it to say that his longtime addiction to chronicle did anything but cooperate with the US Army. Mixing shrewd secretness with open boldness, he obsessively ran roughshod over these military standards to leave us a vivid tale of generals, colonels, doctors, nurses, GIs, POWs, chaplains, everyday people of England, France, Belgium, Luxembourg, and Germany, and himself—all sucked into the vortex of a hospital at war.

More time passed, during which I read even more of the war diaries. That 1983 night in Georgetown and a steady diet of *M*A*S*H* reruns kept me thinking. I could not stop comparing Father John Patrick Francis Mulcahy and what I was glimpsing of Ren as a chaplain, or Colonel Sherman Potter with Ren's commanding officers, or surgeon "Hawkeye" Pierce with any number of Ren's surgeon colleagues, or indeed "Hot Lips" Houlihan with Amy Erickson—a nurse who taught Ren to dance. Striking differences. Also tantalizing similarities. Finally, in 2007, my own life cooperated.

That August I boarded a Delta airplane in Birmingham and headed to Europe for a year of uninterrupted work. My carry-on bag contained that magical "blue box"—an auxiliary hard drive—with digitized copies of Kennedy's correspondence, diaries, and sermons. Because of its central location in the western theater of World War II, Susan, my wife, and I selected the hamlet of Pennedepie in upper Normandy as the home base for our year of tracking Ren Kennedy and the 102nd Evacuation Hospital. However, we also chose Pennedepie because, on an earlier exploratory trip, we had happened upon Marc and Béatrice Ferri. Long-established Parisians, they had a family château in Pennedepie, Val Fontaine—just west of Honfleur—which included a *chaumière* (tiny farmer's cottage) affordable

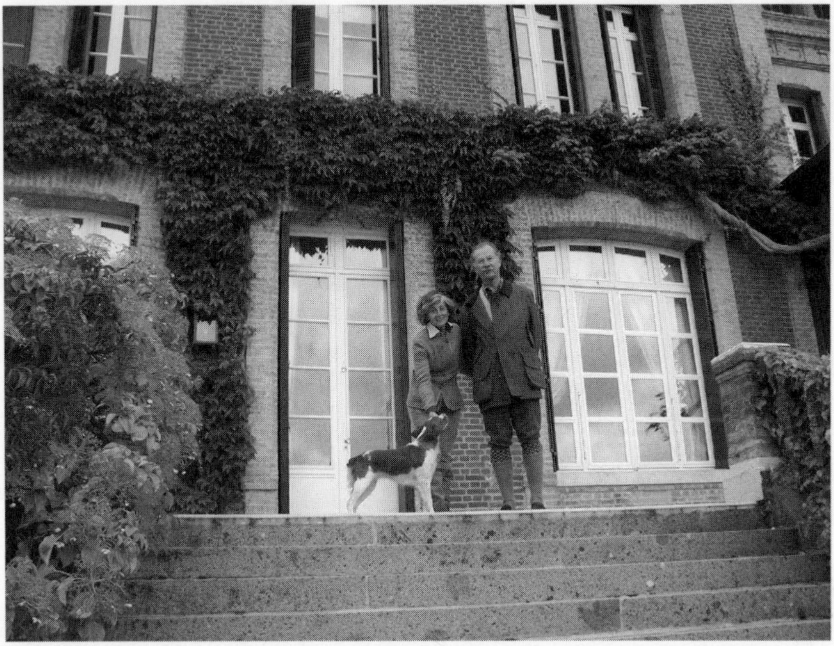

Marc and Béatrice Ferri at Château Val Fontaine. Pennedepie, France (October 2010). Photo by Susan McWilliams.

for a tight budget made even tighter by the exchange rate. We could not have landed better. The whole extended Ferri family treated us like we were theirs. Contrary to American media reports, it was immediately clear that these gracious French people and so many others still had an abiding affection for Americans—if not our current president and vice president and foreign policy—because of what our GIs did for them in World War II.

With each day in Pennedepie I also acquired a stronger appreciation of why that war continued to be so real for the people immediately around us. In 1940 the German SS commandeered the main house of Val Fontaine for its regional headquarters, Marc's father having been sent to prison in Germany for his Resistance leanings while the rest of the family escaped to the south of France. Every morning I walked by this otherwise grand place on the way to my "office"—a studio apartment once the horse attendant's quarters atop a nineteenth-century stable. In my mind's eye I regularly counted the numbers of Mercedes, swastikas, and artillery outside. On numerous evenings Marc and Béatrice treated Susan and me to raw oysters with dry champagne and massive racks of lamb and roasts of pork in the stately dining room where the SS had futilely strategized the defense of Le Havre, just outside the front windows across the mouth of the Seine River. On late afternoon walks with our new and, of course, brilliant Yorkshire terrier, Pennie of Pennedepie, we inspected the hulking bunkers once key to Hitler's Atlantic Wall still punctuating Marc's estate and the neighboring coastline. Rapidly I came to appreciate that the physical manifestations of La Guerre were still powerful components of life in Pennedepie. I saw that for the Ferri family—while never suffering what most Jewish families did—"the war," though ending a half century earlier, remained a tangible, enveloping reality. After a few initial day trips to locations where the 102nd had seen intense action, it also dawned on me that this was the case for virtually all of France and beyond. When laid alongside the unending physical reminders of the war, Ren Kennedy's war writings began to reveal far more detail than I had ever imagined about life inside and outside an evac—and about Ren himself. Indeed, initially using a French map Marc's father had given him, Susan and I began to retrace not just the basic trail of the 102nd through Europe but also every village, schoolhouse, château, and muddy intersection—and virtually every stone wall and pasture and apple orchard—that the 102nd encountered not day by day but hour by hour. Even more, with just a knock on a door and an upbeat "Bonjour," we began to find local citizens eager to help. Here we encountered old people who had detailed remembrances down to specific doctors of "the American tent hospital," especially regarding their efforts to save the lives of "the most innocent of all"—local children. Kennedy's evac diary moved some to raucous laughter, others to stoic analysis, and still others not to words at all—just tears. We also found middle-aged folks whose parents and grandparents had passed down not only concrete recollections but actual documents. One was a diary—long in a desk drawer—recounting how "Captain Kennedy from Alabama sat with us in front of the fire place in the *grand salon* and listened as we talked about German atrocities that ended only as the Americans liberated our village." Regardless of their age, these people embraced Captain Kennedy's chronicles as one more reminder of war's reality and of citizen-soldiers from America who had liberated Europe some fifty years ago. Quickly becoming our friends, they joined the hunt for another compelling episode of World War II.

So, wrought from a multitude of people and places, this is the true story of the 102nd Evacuation Hospital. For me—and for Ren and indeed for any sane human in touch with the personally philosophical nature of war—it also is "the chaplain's conflict."

PART ONE

Finding the War

Even though Susan and I knew we were on the same latitude as Nova Scotia, the rain, the sleet, and the wind of the early fall in Pennedepie caught us off guard. Marc supplied us with a good stock of firewood, and the cottage was cozy—our first experience with an eighteenth-century fireback that propelled the heat well across the tiny living room. Upstairs above the stable I also had Patagonia's best long johns and an electric heater. Yet, whenever I looked up from Ren's writings to gaze out the window upon the whitecaps of the Seine merging with those of the English Channel, it all was less sublime than it was just plain cold. Lots of hot tea.

Actually, after the first hour or so each morning I really didn't look up that much. As that electric heater went to work, how the 102nd organized and trained in California before heading overseas, how people from vastly different backgrounds bonded as a family—with the stresses and strains of virtually all families—captivated me. There was also the personal element of our "inside source" on these developments. Product of a storied South Carolina family and Presbyterian leaders back to the Scottish Reformation, Ren had attended Erskine College—he was classmate and distant kin of the writer Erskine Caldwell—before heading to Princeton Theological Seminary. Accepting the pastorate in south Alabama in 1927, he soon married and started a family. His Wilcox County ministry preceding World War II connected him with the best and the worst in people: courage, humility, and generosity alongside cowardliness, greed, hate, and violence, short of an actual war experience solid preparation for what lay ahead. He also was an avid sports observer—arguably the greatest Crimson Tide football fan ever conceived in South Carolina—and a former high-school athlete still in good shape. He split firewood with the same intensity he played center field at church softball games. Finally, out of modern Christian values, civic duty, and longing for overseas adventure he *wanted* to be in a US Army targeting fascism. Though at forty-three he was exempt from service, he eagerly volunteered and endured six weeks of Victorian-style US Army Chaplain School at Harvard. Still, at that age and with no previous military experience, could he handle a rigorous basic training? Would memories of home with lengthy nocturnal time for reading and writing quickly dilute his intense desire to join the army? Even more, how would his intellectual background shape his observations on a developing evac hospital? That fall in Pennedepie atop Marc's stable Ren began to reveal answers to all this and more.

CHAPTER 1

San Luis Obispo

April–November 1943

On April 9, 1943, Chaplain (First Lieutenant) Kennedy arrived at San Luis Obispo—what military people called "SLO." Originally a California National Guard camp between San Francisco and Los Angeles, in 1943 what Ren encountered was the SLO camp of twenty thousand acres the US Army had recently expanded and modernized for the mobilization of some fifteen thousand personnel attached to wide-ranging armored and infantry units. Created one month before Ren's arrival, the 102nd Evacuation Hospital trained for Pacific action as part of the II Armored Corps. Immediately he attended an orientation meeting with his CO, Lt. Col. Carlton D. Goodiel, a World War I veteran and career army physician two years his senior. He found that the 102nd had some thirty physicians, fifteen staff officers, and 250 enlisted men. The "men," however, were more likely boys, March 1943 draftees chiefly from Arkansas, Oklahoma, and Texas, most with high-school educations. The unit's thirty female nurses—members of the new US Army Nursing Corps—would join the unit after basic training. He also found that his "flock," for the time being, was anything but a heavy load by World War II chaplaincy standards.

At that time, at least, it consisted of whatever basic-training patients there were from throughout the SLO camp (at least three other evacs were there as well) and the 102nd's regular 325 personnel, who were 24 percent Catholic, 2 percent Jewish, and 74 percent Protestant. Just as he had been instructed at the Harvard chaplain school, at services he was to reflect the theology of his own personal "faith group"—generic Protestant. The large number of Catholic chaplains in the army and the tiny number of Jewish chaplains would do the generic same. Moreover, his faith-group message was to be just that—not the army's. The army had no theology per se. As for non-Protestants in his developing flock, he was to give them appropriate prayer books and facilitate their services with Jewish or Catholic

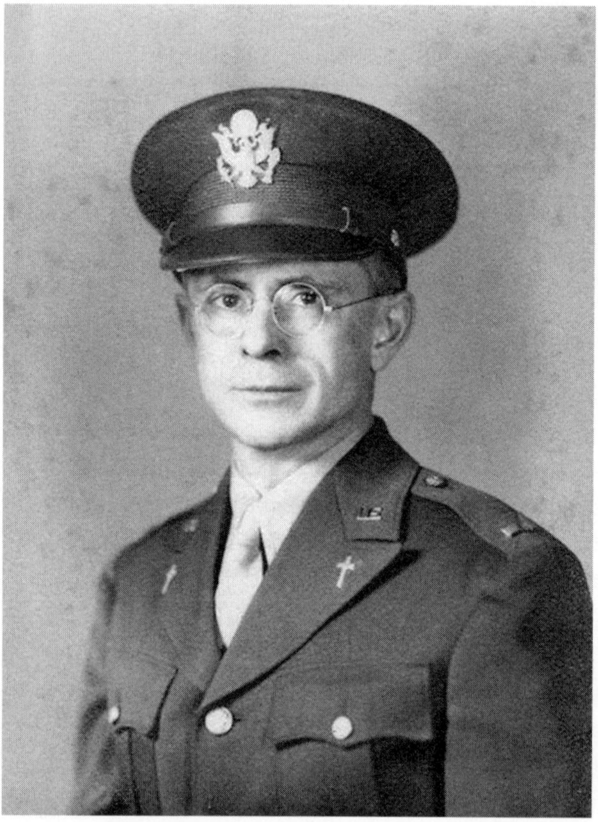

RCK upon graduation from US Army Chaplain School at Harvard, Cambridge, Massachusetts (March 1943). US Army photo in RCK Papers.

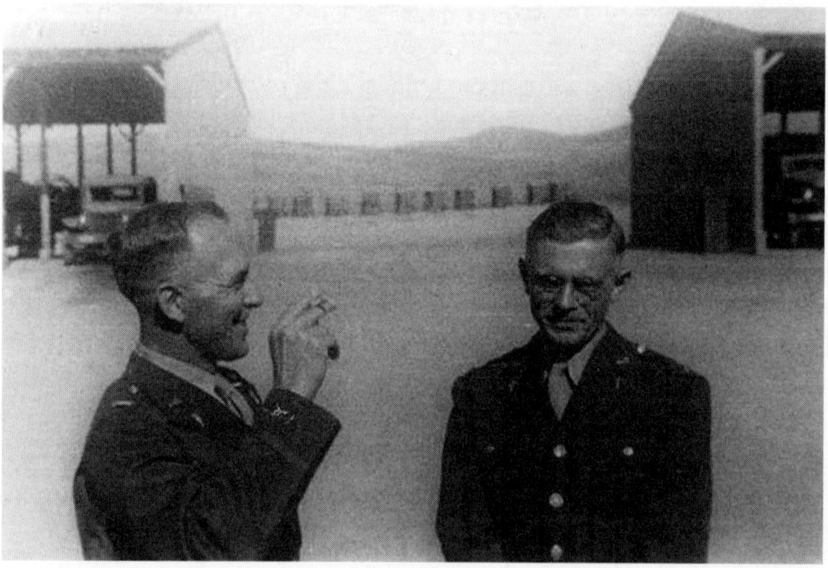

Lt. Col. Carleton D. Goodiel (left), initial CO of the 102nd Evacuation Hospital, and RCK. San Luis Obispo, California, April 1943. Unknown photographer. RCK Papers.

chaplains. He savored the ecumenical sound of all this, especially its lack of Protestant denominationalism.

Settled into his "hutment" with Tennessee roommate 1st Lt. Daniel M. Laws and into an office in the nearby HQ tent, Ren found the succeeding eight months at SLO for the most part predictable, useful, and enjoyable. An average weekday in camp had him visiting "the boys" in the wards. As per army requirements, at least once a week after lunch he gave a "sexual morality" lecture. Some thirty "men and boys" normally showed up—no doctors. A non-Victorian on sex and one who understood the army's practical concerns about overly active sex lives increasing chances for sexually transmitted diseases and reducing the army's effectiveness, he realistically urged responsibility (rather than abstinence), plus the wrongness of "taking advantage of young girls who will approach you." More to his liking, he attended what he called "Army doctor seminars" on chemical warfare, basics of army field medicine, symptoms of true battle fatigue, new techniques in abdominal surgery, and the use of Benzedrine pills to stay awake. He also embraced all physical training, including long marches in the rain with a forty-pound pack and indeed obstacle courses with barbed wire and live ammunition fired overhead. Considered noncombatants by both the Geneva Convention and army policy, army chaplains were not to carry even sidearms in combat but had the option for firearms training should combat bring them into unanticipated defensive situations. A crack-shot quail hunter in early years and one comfortable with firearms in his home, Ren opted for both M1 rifle and .45-cal. pistol training.

To "stay in touch" he split his meals between the officers' mess and the men's mess. After supper he "counseled" anyone with a problem who cared to drop in—occasionally physicians, more often "the boys." Still in the office from around 10:00 PM to 11:00 PM he used a treasured army-issue Remington portable typewriter to file untreasured army chaplaincy reports and respond to the steady stream of letters from his wife, Mary, and his two daughters, Mary Conway, fourteen, and Margaret, eleven, and from congregation members. Long a nocturnal creature, he concluded most SLO nights about 12:30 AM with twenty minutes in his diary, bedtime noted often after waking roommate Laws for "the precise time" since the Lathan military watch he bought at chaplain school kept losing time—"at least a minute a day, more or less." Once every two weeks the entire 102nd Evacuation Hospital packed up and moved out in trucks and Jeeps for overnight bivouacs to train in just that—transporting the hospital—and also in admitting and treating simulated casualties in the

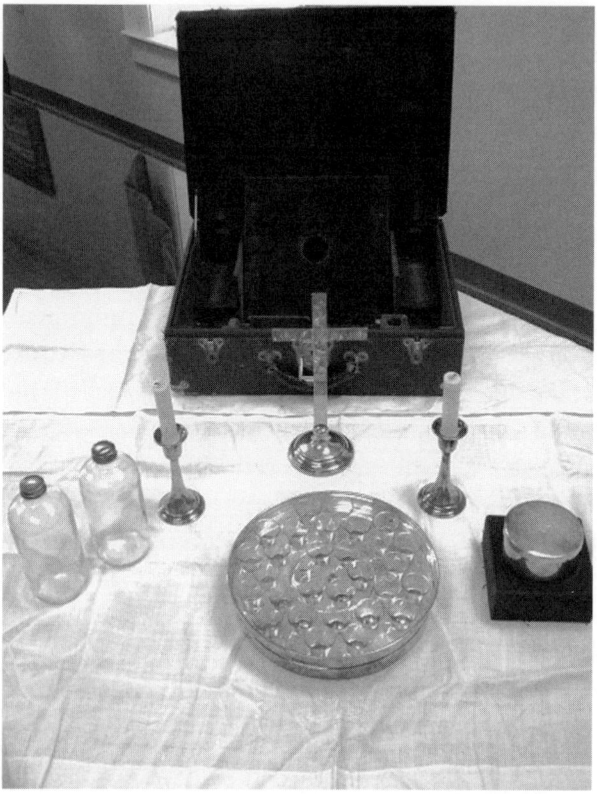

RCK's field communion kit, provided by the Presbyterian (PCUSA) Committee on Camp Activities. Courtesy Haas Strother, Camden, Alabama; photo, August 2011, by Mary Ann Wright.

field. Ren never missed a bivouac, often traveling by Jeep with CO Goodiel or the chief of surgery, Arthur A. Sutherland.

Then there were Sundays. At 10:00 AM, with the help of a "chaplain assistant," a Seventh Day Adventist and conscientious objector from Freeport, Maine, named Roland Rhynus, Ren regularly delivered a service in the 102nd's recreation hall, using a portable altar, communion field kit, and cross, all of which he had to "acquire" through the Presbyterian (PCUSA) Committee on Camp Activities. Attuned as he was to army guidelines, the sermons reflected his personal, Protestant wartime concerns: the need for Americans to have humility in the current conflict, Germany's rejection of God, and why going to war was a necessary sin in a Christian context. At 1:30 PM Ren repeated the sermon in the guardhouse for the fifteen to twenty usually incarcerated—"100% attendance" normally guaranteed by cigarettes all around, complimentary of the ever-smoking (pipe, cigarettes, sometimes cigars) chaplain. He then spent late afternoons in his room napping and reading before opening up the office for Sunday night counseling.

Ren's counseling at SLO harkened back to life in Alabama while foreshadowing what lay ahead overseas. It was everyday "social issues" intensified by a military, if technically noncombat, environment. Standard fare included AWOL, venereal disease, Red Cross contacts for travel money home upon a death in the family, and soldiers' stealing from other soldiers. Theft usually involved money, but valued articles were taken, too. Indeed, when an ordinance officer lifted Ren's own Remington typewriter, he recovered it only after a special counseling session with executive officer Edward K. Prigge. Less common was a meeting with a soldier who raped the visiting wife of another soldier and the counseling of soldier friends of three "boys" who died in the 102nd hospital at SLO, one from a Jeep wreck, one from an M1 rifle accident, and the other from an apparent allergic reaction to morphine. Counseling could also bring him humor: the case of two soldiers who got badly drunk off base, only to be arrested by two MPs who were also drunk, and on return to camp the soldiers' protesting they could drive more effectively than the MPs, causing the Jeep to wreck, with the related chaos of broken arms and legs. The most popular topic of all, however, was "How can I get out of the Army?" Ren attributed the majority of these would-be "exiters" to either physicians who saw lucrative practices slipping away while they were in the military or the makeup of the enlisted portion of the 102nd, overwhelmingly nineteen to twenty-year-old boys from rural backgrounds who, before the army, had "never spent more than a few nights away from home in their lives." Some "homesick" cases evolved to bed-wetting or crying, accompanied by public ostracism; three of these led to self-shooting in an arm or a leg. However, "get[ting] out of the Army" was not that easy. In the 102nd, even if Ren's initial interview concluded that an "exiter needed to go," a physician had to authorize a Certificate of Disability Discharge (CDD), which then had to have CO approval. At SLO apparently two extreme homesickness cases in the 102nd departed—both for "nervous complaint (crying)." Two other cases did, too. One drafted private who was ostracized for his homosexuality and was open in discussing it with Ren left on a mandatory CDD, which was consistent with army policy at that time, although not without debate among Ren (whose Alabama friends included several homosexuals) and a few physicians about the army's position on "tolerance" and its uses of "disability." A "boy from

Arkansas" who had not completed the second grade and could neither read nor write—"cruel, never should have been drafted"—had no clue as to the content of the training manuals "on guns or marching or anything." Ren facilitated the necessary CDD. After this second departure Ren sought CO approval for establishing correspondence courses on literacy for soldiers who were "borderline on reading and writing." He also sought a small discretionary "chaplain's fund," through which he might hire soldiers to act as tutors. When both efforts went nowhere, he and "a sergeant" tried their best to serve as volunteer tutors.

Ren's concerns about literacy were part of a broader preoccupation with the human mind in the 102nd Evacuation Hospital. He found surprisingly few "intellectuals in the outfit." Among his close 102nd friends at SLO, only the chief of medicine, James J. Barfield, and Adjutant Joseph Rutenberg read something other than "an occasional *Reader's Digest*." Although an intense sports fan—not just a football fan but also a careful analyst of major league baseball and Joe Louis's fights—Ren lamented that, even with the Allied invasion of Italy, most of the surgeons read only "the sports page and maybe the funny papers" in the *Los Angeles Times,* leaving "the rest of the paper untouched." He regularly read the *Los Angeles Times* (delivered to his office door) and the *New Republic* and *Christian Century* (mailed subscriptions). When he offered to share particularly interesting articles with the doctors and other officers, he had no takers. Lack of ideas merged with "low morale" to deliver more than a few "tight, tense days." He attributed this in great part to the "narrowness" of senior leadership, carried over from the peacetime army. A colonel visiting the 102nd "bawled out" Dan Laws, whose duties as first lieutenant included responsibility for the mess halls, when the colonel discovered "a mop" left out of place. The episode reminded Ren of a career army officer he had encountered in the Harvard program who advised Ren that he should plan to spend "at least two hours out of every day" making sure his uniform was in order—"screwy . . . anything that requires that." Similarly, older senior officers at SLO—colonels and above, including his CO, Goodiel—were not as interested in why the United States needed to win the war as they were with "petty matters of possibly peace time consequence only." With no consistently focused directive from the top, as Ren saw it, the lesser officers (not to mention the nonofficers) tended to wallow in their own preoccupations. On departing Wilcox County, Alabama, Ren had hoped for "a bigger Army."

Still, for Ren these daily frustrations were more than offset by myriad SLO adventures. He bonded with many—although it took several months at SLO for these bonds to move him beyond the military habit of calling buddies by their last names. He relished the nighttime bivouac parties out in the field with the army funding the refreshments—"64 gallons of beer, 290 packages of cigarettes"—where soldiers of all ranks could talk about daily life. "Our boys do a lot of hard work." Still, his close friends clearly came from the officer ranks. Saturday afternoons normally found Ren golfing at the nearby Moro Beach course with his regular partner, Dan Laws. Raised a Southern Baptist in Elizabethton, Tennessee, Laws at age twenty-four had just graduated from East Tennessee State College and been accepted by the University of Virginia law school when the war called. Despite being some twenty years older, Ren thrived in the regular company of this smart, mildly raucous former college football player. Laws's initial experience with higher education ended when Carson-Newman College expelled him for force-shaving a freshman's head. Their instantly close friendship launched them into golf and many other wartime adventures.

Ren's other golfing regulars included surgeon William P. Jennings, Detachment Commander Joseph Rutenberg, Adjutant Basil M. Winstead, Warrant Officer Clarence H. ("Woojie") Schmittdiel, and dentist Lee H. Montgomery. He thought about the elitist role golf could play in general society; he even noted in the diary certain caustic lines from a Sara Hopkins poem: "The golf links lie so near the mill that almost everyday the laboring children can look out and see the men at play." But he relished golf anyhow. He bought clubs and showed little of the frustration that most neophyte golfers exhibited. For eighteen holes it was "108 today . . . an enjoyable day."

Saturday nights saw the golfers drinking and dining at Mattie's Place on Pismo Bay or at off-base apartments that a few officers rented for their wives. The Laws's apartment, despite newborn baby—Ren baptized Daniel M. Laws III—held special status for "east Tennessee-style" fried chicken. On still other Saturday nights he enjoyed promotion parties. Here were blowout gatherings jointly funded by promoted individuals and open to all officers of the 102nd, with consumption of copious amounts of Lucky Lager beer, countless Lucky Strike cigarettes, and sometimes hard liquor. His discrete cocktailing in Wilcox County gave way to alcohol without a shroud. Still, in the diary he often noted which of his good new friends got drunk, when the army should have been more restrained with regard to alcohol ("Division reception—punch had to have been nearly straight gin"), and even those apparently isolated times when he drank too much. "HQ dance tonight . . . bored . . . get too many slugs." Too, he rarely passed up division softball games, whether in the stands or playing centerfield, or hutment gatherings with Laws, Sutherland, and others for penny poker and canasta with innovative alcohol—"slugs of rum and brandy, interesting." Usually accompanied by Dan and Gladys Laws, he also took advantage of notables hosted by the camp or the division, like Bob Hope, Joe Louis, Jackie Robinson, Rudee Vallée, and Sugar Ray Robinson, and first-run films: Lena Horne and Cab Calloway in *Stormy Weather* ("very good"), Henry Fonda in *The Oxbow Incident* ("good"), Bette Davis in *Watch on the Rhine* ("good"), Roy Rogers in *Hands across the Border* ("sorry").

Even more, beginning a pattern soon to carry him on a "trans-oceanic tour," he never missed an opportunity to savor the surrounding nonarmy scene. When a Presbyterian minister from the community of SLO, Frederick J. Hart, invited him to the home of "a Mrs. Richards" for a night of listening to phonograph recordings of Richard Wagner with commentary by the hostess, Ren jumped at the opportunity. When a black chaplain from Memphis, Samuel A. Owen, a senior career officer based at SLO, mentioned that a steer-riding rodeo was about to occur at nearby California Polytechnic Institute, off they went in a "borrowed" Jeep facilitated by Laws and accompanied by another SLO chaplain, Catholic priest William A. Molyneux. For Thanksgiving leave he drove cross-country with Basil Winstead in his 1941 Plymouth through the Mojave Desert and the lower Grand Canyon ("magnificent scenery!"), then on to Little Rock before taking a Benzedrine pill and training down to Camden. In terms of sheer geography, however, the bivouacs of the 102nd gave Ren his "greatest views": the Big Sur Mountains, the Pacific Ocean, the Hearst Palace. After Lieutenant Colonel Goodiel asked Ren to ride out with him for a day through the Salinas Valley and Monterey to inspect a site for an upcoming bivouac, Ren immersed himself in John Steinbeck's fictional depiction of that area, *Tortilla Flat*—available at the camp library, "which no one ever [went] to." His trips were "fascinating" and "beautiful." He hungered for adventures to accompany army life. At SLO the 102nd Evacuation Hospital more than provided those thrills.

CHAPTER 2

Goffs

December 1943–February 1944

In October 1943 the 102nd Evacuation Hospital found itself refocused. Instead of the Pacific, it would head for the European theater. To at least partially prepare it for duty in a rough European winter—significant foresight—on December 3, 1943, the US Army sent the 102nd to icy, windblown Goffs, California, some four hundred miles east in the Mohave Desert. It was not the anticipated four months of simulated battle and frigid tents that made Ren "hate to leave [the] home" of SLO, as he wrote Mary. Despite its "morale issues" he had bonded with the unit in the liberated, exciting environment of SLO. San Luis Obispo *was* home. Yet it turned out that "home" just moved with him. If Goffs was "desolate" and "icy with rain," "no morning shave unless you melt the ice," "Dan and I" still roomed together, along with three other officers, in a tent that had an oil stove and a wooden floor. Lee Montgomery transferred out of the 102nd, but the newly minted Birmingham anesthesiologist, Capt. Edward Peterson, joined the unit and became another close Alabama friend sharing Ren's fascination with the Santa Fe trains that were hurtling down the tracks adjacent to Goffs.

Ren's Sunday services continued in the men's mess tent, his counseling in a one-man pup tent with a desk and two chairs. After just four days at Goffs he wrote Mary, "It's going to be an interesting experience. I am going to enjoy it." In fact, two days later, on Thursday, December 9, Ren received notice of his promotion to captain retroactive to November 20. He wrote Mary, "From now on you will please address me as Captain . . . $50 a month more pay. . . . [Mary now] had $200 a month which is as much [as] or more than all four of us had to live on." With captain's bars a joint gift from Dan Laws and Joe Rutenberg, Ren gleefully organized the customary promotion party for the officers of the 102nd "in [the] recreation tent, 60 bottles of beer, 25 coca colas, 50 cigars, 20 candy bars, pretzels, cheese, peanuts, chewing gum." The event must have been "underwritten" by Dan Laws's selectively guarded quartermaster supplies, for the host's total personal costs—at least what he told his wife—were "$12 or $13," and he was "glad to spend it."

Promotion did not dampen Ren's intensity about the physical aspects of army life. Although most of his captain colleagues who were physicians dodged the intensified obstacle courses with live fire whistling overhead and the simulated battle in the sleet, Ren took on these "trying conditions" and told Mary he was "doing ok with it all" and "enjoying it." Still, the intentionally rougher training at Goffs significantly expanded his workload. More and more of the "boys," as well as nonmedical officers from throughout the Goffs operations, were seriously hurt in accidents with grenades and live ammunition. By mid-December, despite theoretically being in training, the tent wards of the 102nd had two hundred beds filled with "true battle type cases." By late December there were three hundred, "more patients than all three hospitals in Selma [Alabama] can handle." For the first time Ren was consistently doing heavy bedside counseling in the wards. To facilitate these sessions he strategically expanded his knowledge of surgery by "observing" various procedures still under way after he closed his evening office counseling. Likewise, he found the newly arrived nursing component of the 102nd—thirty of them—filled with talented caregivers and good instructors on what patients had what odds for certain recoveries. Most of the nurses he thus met became friends, and they seemed more interested in his Sunday services in the recreation tent than others did, notably "three Jewish nurses" who regularly sat beside his close friends Basil Winstead and Joe Rutenberg, who were also Jewish.

In "honor" of Ren's promotion, CO Goodiel asked Captain Kennedy to supervise the plans for the Christmas celebration. Ren enjoyed the additional assignment of coordinating with the Red Cross, and on Christmas day small gift packages valued at $1.00 each—a combination of socks, chewing gum, toothbrushes, shaving cream, or Jergens lotion—went to all of the patients and every member of the 102nd, a labor-intensive project in which Ren received much "assigned help" from the nurses. The venture required several trips to Pasadena to procure the needed supplies, permitting him to drop off that vexing Lathan military watch at Edleman's, where it was finally "fixed." Increasingly aware that a chaplain's duties were "varied" (he had private whiskey orders for Laws, Barfield, and Sutherland), much as a nurse's were, while in Pasadena Ren and his truck driver had to pick up furniture for Goodiel's newly rented home at Goffs—no tent life for the CO, which for Ren bode poorly for "morale problems."

Still, Christmas "was the most remarkable [he] ever had.... Packed and jammed [in the recreation tent on Christmas Eve] I could not count them all... [Then] Xmas carols in front of each ward tent... 50 people [singing], even some patients came out and joined. SGT Roy Thraikell brought his bugle out and blew the music for every song." This exuberance continued on Christmas Day. Ren, the self-proclaimed intellectual, served as Santa. Assisted by Roland Rhynus, he handed out gift boxes under "gigantic" trees in the men's and the officers' messes before individually visiting the three hundred patients in the ward tents and finally presiding over "turkey Christmas dinners in shifts." "Tired" and "with head ache" but certain it was "a good day," that night in his tent Ren had slugs and opened packages from home. He was so preoccupied with Dan's coveting his favorite gift—shelled pecans from his younger sister Margaret in South Carolina—that he managed to write only a short letter to Mary ("It was certainly the busiest Christmas I have ever had") before turning in at 1:00 AM. The next day the larger reality intruded. "I don't know about next Xmas," he wrote Mary, "but certainly I hope to spend Xmas of 1945 with you and the children."

Despite an uplifting Christmas, the winter of 1942–1943 saw morale problems worsen under weak senior leadership. When the 102nd had a day or so with few beds occupied, most of the unit went out on crucially complicated load/unload/set up exercises. Many of the physician officers, however, "elected" to stay in camp or "just take the day off," and some of them got "badly drunk." However, CO Goodiel took no steps to remedy this lack of discipline, which could seriously compromise the unit in actual combat. Goodiel himself even "took off" during some of these exercises. "The men" increasingly went to Ren to protest the unfairness and ineffectiveness of the situation. In turn, wondering how Goodiel "could get away with this," Ren repeatedly took the matter to Executive Officer Ed Prigge ("a fine man... far superior to the Colonel"), who was equally frustrated with the CO. Prigge theorized that Goodiel's unwillingness to back him up on officer discipline was a strategy the CO pursued to get low efficiency ratings and thereby keep himself from being sent into action overseas.

Just as disconcerting was Goodiel's refusal to address the nurses' "hatred" of the chief of nursing, 1st Lt. Frances Ewing. Here, as Ren wrote Mary, was a "mean and selfish woman," "a genuine battle axe," and "just a very unhappy person" who took out her unhappiness on the nurses by only criticizing, never praising. Individually and in small groups the nurses came to Ren for guidance on how to coexist with Ewing; he discussed the problem with the ever-frustrated Prigge and on a Jeep ride also raised the issue with Goodiel. When nothing happened, in his office he personally talked with Ewing about easing up on her personnel. Although he tried to get the conversation off to a happy start with "hot rum and tea," things rapidly deteriorated, he told Mary, and he had to "jolt her once or twice with verbal jabs," which led to Ewing's threatening to bar her nurses from "going to church." This did not happen. However, Ren saw the prospects of it as movement toward "open warfare."

Even when the physicians—whom Goodiel normally coddled—complained to the CO that the nurses' morale was so low due to Ewing that their effectiveness in the wards had been reduced and that she was "a thorn in the flesh of practically everyone in the outfit," nothing occurred—except that in late February 1944 Ewing found herself promoted to captain. That was all that Executive Officer Prigge could take. Goodiel approved his transfer out, which brought Ren into his highest-stake crisis counseling so far. As he told his diary, nurses and physicians had pleaded with him to advise Goodiel that "No one wants Sutherland to become executive officer [replacing Prigge] . . . [because he] is loud and vulgar . . . nor [William] Stewart to succeed him as chief of surgery." Although he told Goodiel this, both of them nonetheless moved up. Ren liked Sutherland—they were poker partners—but he still viewed these disconcerting developments as further evidence of a big flaw among the seniormost officers. "I have yet to meet one person [among the key decision makers] of first-class ability and personal qualities who belongs to the regular Army. . . . This is a civilian Army, and it is civilians who are doing the job."

Indeed, the intensified training at Goffs and the resultant influx of seriously hurt soldiers led to Ren's expanded experience with one particular type of citizen-soldier—the black soldier. Much of army life in 1944 remained as legally segregated as everyday life in Alabama. The army generally restricted black soldiers to all-black ordinance and motor-pool endeavors. Still, the wall of discrimination in the army had both intentional and unintentional cracks of flexibility, and from life in Wilcox County Ren understood what this allowed. At Harvard he seemed fully at ease with the army's 1942 decision to desegregate its chaplain-training program, which predated the general desegregation of the US military by six years. At SLO he saw the irony that the army had white soldiers in one truck and Negro soldiers in another, yet through happenstance on one occasion, "in the rain the Negro soldiers have a canopy over them" while the white soldiers did not. He also enjoyed the freedom he had for at least some interracial social life with fellow black chaplains at SLO—the rodeo trip with Chaplain Owen—despite the fact that black chaplains were assigned to "Negro units." So by the time he got to Goffs he perceived no oddity when the otherwise segregated army sent black soldiers to the 102nd to be cared for in interracial wards. Indeed, black soldiers of the 93rd Infantry Division, as one of the few black combat units in the army (soon to be active in the Pacific theater), trained twenty miles from Goffs at Camp Clipper and were among those badly hurt in the risky desert exercises. In late December 1943 "half of our [three hundred] patients are Negroes from the 93rd," he told his diary, pleased that many who could walk attended his services, where they showed "greater interests in receiving the Testaments" he distributed than the white soldiers did. "Negroes" were also part of the "fine service" he had on Christmas Eve and among the many he visited in the beds.

Most of the patients from the 93rd had standard counseling issues (e.g., "a Negro patient" whose hands had been injured "got me to write letters to [his] Lt. to collect debts for him on pay day" since he was in the hospital). However, of all the patients he visited before he went to Europe, none engaged Ren more than a platoon leader with the 93rd, 1st Lt. Vasco D. Hale from Fairmont, West Virginia. With no counseling appointments on the night of December 30, Ren went to the wards early to watch the surgeries. He had already witnessed "a bloody night in our hospital" involving others from the 93rd when an ambulance delivered Hale. The following night he wrote Mary:

> Lt. Hale . . . had been injured by an explosion of hand-grenades. . . . They gave him shock treatment for a few hours, blood plasma, glucose [then] started to work on him about 11 PM. They finished at 3:00 AM. Capt [Lawrence] Dickey did the surgery. Capt. [Douglas] Dodge helped, and Capt [?] gave the anesthetic. . . . They had to remove one arm below the

> elbow, and the other hand. Both of his eyes were blown out and his face [was] mangled.... It was a long and bloody job picking the metal and dirt out of his face.... Tonight [New Year's Eve] I talked with him some. His whole head is bandaged except for his mouth. He kept saying, 'I can't see,' and repeated, 'Holy, Holy, Lord God.'... I told him his face was wrapped up. He said, 'I couldn't see before they wrapped it up. I won't ever see.'... He wanted to know if his wife had been notified. I went to the registrar's tent and found that she had been sent a telegram. I told him. He wanted to know where they sent it. It was sent to his home in West Virginia. He said his wife was not there, was in Cleveland at Western Reserve University. So I had the clerk in the registrar's tent send another telegram to her. He said he and his wife corresponded a great deal and she would know something was wrong by not hearing from him. He has certainly been fine and brave about it. The doctors say he may not live.

On New Year's day the 102nd evacuated Lieutenant Hale to a general hospital. After seeing him off in the ambulance, Ren wrote Mary, "I see a lot of sad and tragic things." (Defying predictions, Hale—before the war a noted athlete, graduate of West Virginia State College, and a revered high school biology teacher—lived for some sixty years, storied for his leadership with the NAACP and veterans' groups despite being blind, deaf, and paraplegic.) Long sensitive to courage in everyday lives, Ren nevertheless moved on with a deeper notion of adventure in wartime, viewing Hale as "so much dignity regardless of the horror."

Despite morale issues and "sad things"—perhaps in part because of them—as January and February 1944 unfolded Ren looked upon the 102nd even more as "home." In late January rumors began circulating that deployment to Europe was fast approaching. The CO approved Ren for a ten-day "good-bye" home leave. Ren and Ed Peterson drove to Alabama in the physician's white 1940 Chevrolet convertible, "top not down." From the camp's Special Services tent he brought daughter Mary Conway a copy of *Tortilla Flat,* intended as a "give-away for the soldiers but the men ... prefer comic books." On Sunday, January 30, he preached at three different churches in Wilcox County—the Christian obligation to defeat fascism alongside basic-training adventure stories. He also had the hands of his Lathan watch further adjusted at Bewigs in Selma so that at "12 noon both hands are precisely on the twelve"—"a precise wrist watch is such a convenient thing to have"—though it still continued to "gain a little."

On February 18 the uplifting elements of Goffs life resumed as Ren, Dan, and Joe Rutenberg grabbed time to visit Boulder Dam and Las Vegas ("wide open . . . gambling is legal . . . everything else too"), and on his return Ren wrote Mary, "I have more or less fallen in love with the desert . . . very beautiful" with flowers and cactus. In the Special Services tent he came upon a copy of Honoré Balzac's perverse short story, "A Passion in the Desert," keeping a key line for the diary: The desert is "'God without mankind.'" Even an otherwise wretched blustery day in camp merited "it is very nice to hear the [rain] on the tent at night." As for the people and the patients of the 102nd, "we have our problems," he confided to Mary, but "I have come to feel about these men pretty much about the way I did about the members of my own church."

On February 21 Goodiel announced that the 102nd would be moving "east" within ten days to prepare for the Atlantic crossing. Once their Goffs camp began to close, no member of the 102nd could communicate about cross-country travel schedules or subsequent departure plans. Thrilled, as a longtime connoisseur of good mystery novels, as well as symbolism based on local flora, Ren immediately suggested to Mary that they should have their "own code": "When I write you that the Ocotillo cactus are in bloom that will mean it is my last letter" upon leaving Goffs. On March 6 Goodiel confided to Ren that they would go by train to New York City, then on to neighboring Camp Kilmer in New Jersey in preparation for boarding ship. When writing Mary, Ren dutifully withheld this information and said only, "I don't mind going . . . except being so far from you and the children." He also told her he would mail Conway an army copy ("no compunctions of conscience") of Joseph Conrad's *Lord Jim*. Yet he so much looked "forward . . . to what is ahead" that on Wednesday, March 8, the day before leaving Goffs, he ran right over his own secret code. "The Ocotillo cactus is blooming," he carefully advised Mary. "We go to New York." The censors missed it.

CHAPTER 3

New York to Southport

March–July 1944

After four days on the rails the eleven cars of the 102nd unloaded at Penn Station, then trucked across the Hudson River twenty miles to New Jersey's Camp Kilmer, recently constructed by the army as a major transition point for troops heading overseas. Two weeks of "hurry up and wait" ensued. The troops undertook one long march in the rain, listened to lectures on boarding and "deboarding" a ship made more than bearable by regular barracks ("real beds and real food"), and were granted leaves to New York City. During the cross-country trip and the Camp Kilmer stay Ren never missed offering a Sunday service. But in New York City his intensity shifted. Mary visited. She and Ren, along with Dan and Gladys Laws, enjoyed a three-hour dinner and floor show ("$9.00 a couple") at Jack Dempsey's club. The next day the Kennedys caught Anton Chekhov's *Cherry Orchard* at the National Theater ("Eva Le Gallien [*sic*] and Joseph Schieldkrut . . . fine acting"), then ate broiled flounder while watching ice skaters at Rockefeller Center. When the wives departed, Ren sought to take Dan out to Princeton to see his old haunts, but constant rain steered them instead toward repeated stops for "six short beers" in Manhattan—conservative compared to one physician's self-reported record of "57 glasses of beer in twelve hours." Despite "extraordinary drinking and drunks around me," leaving the "memory" of the 102nd "befogged," Ren managed to protect his private time. Normally one to read literature related to where he was, he managed to forego the paltry poem "Trees," written by the man whose name and monument adorned their camp, "poet-soldier" of World War I—Joyce Kilmer. Instead, he read Philip Stong's novel *State Fair.* On March 29 he returned to the city to see Paul Robeson and José Ferrer in William Shakespeare's *Othello.* Then it was over.

On April 6, 1944, the 102nd Evacuation Hospital, in its own particular "fog," departed New York harbor with other soldiers on the five-hundred-foot "antique" *RMS Tamaroa* as part of a thirty-ship convoy headed to

England. With four hundred hammocks on board, the two thousand GIs slept in shifts. For his first time at sea Ren had it better. As chief (and only) ship's chaplain, with additional duties of being the special services officer (Red Cross liaison, dispenser of free cigarettes, director of a pick-up quartet though he could not carry a tune), he shared a stateroom with Dan and two other officers. On Friday evening, April 7, he coordinated Jewish services with a Jewish enlisted man conducting. On April 9 a "beautiful Easter Sunday" unfolded on the open ocean. He coordinated two Catholic "services" (without Mass) with the aid of a Catholic enlisted man and preached seven Protestant Communion services between 9:30 AM and 2:45 PM in the holds, the lounges, and the "brig (17 on hand)" to a total of 758 before recovering that afternoon with a dinner of poached sea bass. No slugs on board—rigidly enforced. April 12, however, brought the start of a three-day storm, in which "2 men [were] lost overboard," and the nights were made doubly dangerous by "running without lights" to avoid German submarine attacks. At least once during the storm an accompanying destroyer had to fend off U-boats with depth charges. "Without lights" meant not even smoking a cigarette on deck. Ren shuttered as some still lit up before being ushered to the brig: "I see it. . . . [They] risk 2000 people for a smoke."

After eleven days at sea the *Tamaroa* sighted Ireland. "Going around the w. coast of Ireland . . . convoy [a] beautiful sight . . . [with] fore and aft lights burning." As the 102nd approached Avonmouth, England (near Bristol), on the Irish Sea, he wrote Mary "from somewhere in England"—as army censors required—that he "enjoyed the trip." In further conformity with the censors' regulations he omitted mentioning the casualties during the storm and the genuine possibility that the entire ship could have gone down with one well-placed torpedo. He focused instead on his satisfaction with the Easter services at sea.

On Wednesday, April 19, the 102nd departed Bristol by train for the twelve-hour ride north to Southport, also on the Irish Sea (near Liverpool), where other US Army units were located alongside various components of the London government seeking refuge from the German bombs. At least six of the 102nd's forty officers—those sharing a compartment with Ren—rode that train to Southport drunk on "medical alcohol" stolen from the *Tamaroa*'s hospital and exited the train in the same condition. The chaplain clearly was discovering how "medical alcohol" fit into the evac life. For the time being, however, he was only too happy just to survive the train ride and land securely in the conservative

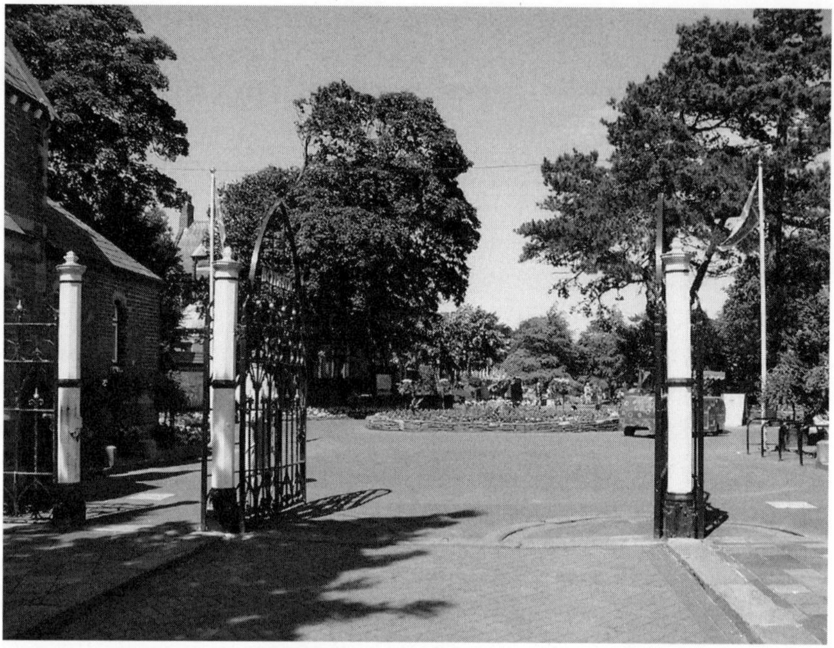

The botanical gardens in Southport, England, where the 102nd established general operations during the summer of 1944, awaiting the "crossover" (October 2010). Photo courtesy of Margaret Delaney, Crosby, England.

home of Raymond and Margaret Garton, 21 Preston New Road, in the adjacent village of Churchtown, where he individually billeted—a four-minute train ride into Southport but, weather permitting, a "most pleasant" thirty-minute walk. "A fine man," Raymond Garton had worked for the same sawmill in Hull for fifty-four years, starting out as an office boy and winding up a regional salesman before German bombs destroyed the mill—and his job—in May of 1941. Although they "had some savings" and a home, the Gartons' "income" was the billeting fee paid by the US Army. In their stucco cottage Ren had one of the two bedrooms. It came equipped with "heavy . . . complete and thorough . . . blackout curtains," and he shared the single bathroom with the Gartons. Although he took his meals in the 102nd's mess, set up along with their other general operations in the Southport Botanical Gardens, every night that he was "home" he joined the Gartons for tea and cakes at 10:00 PM in front of a small coal fire, where he and Raymond listened (Mrs. Garton was "stone deaf") to the war news on the radio before "black out curtains at 10:15 PM." Ren in turn bought them candy, soap, and pipe tobacco at the Southport PX and had their rarest and most valued commodity—tea—mailed from Wilcox County, Alabama, compliments of Mary.

With life in a private home, no more live-fire obstacle courses, and the 102nd evac hospital packed and awaiting orders, Ren's normal workday in England was anything but taxing. Sunday services usually unfolded outdoors at the Southport Botanical Gardens. On perhaps half of these Sundays he went directly from the 102nd's morning service to deliver "a guest sermon" at neighboring Methodist, Anglican, Congregational, or Presbyterian churches—an army request that was "good" for community relations. On some weekday mornings there were general marches—nurses included—but on most days Ren went to the gardens with other officers for classes ranging from conversational German and French, to aircraft identification, to "unending" analyses of army organization. In the afternoons he continued with counseling services in an office at the 102nd's HQ, established in the Florentine-style Bold Hotel on Lord Street. Two blocks from the Bold, inside the massive two-hundred-year-old city hall and courthouse building, the officers of the 102nd had a club, where Ren devoted many "off hours." Here he enjoyed "my new sport" (ping-pong) and followed the war news on the radio. Here, too, was regular consumption of Guinness stout beer with Dan and physician friends. One doctor showed him how to "mix two bottles of Guinness and a light beer . . . [a] mix [that] is called locally a 'black and tan.'" Although the army had to recall two of these 102nd physicians from Southport to the States because of alcohol problems, Ren still "liked both of them."

Out of all of this "normal-day" activity a French class occasionally caught his attention, as did "a black and white shaggy puppy" he "met" on a march. So did counseling problems. A particular one stood out. Commanding Officer Goodiel received a letter from a woman in Southport who was angry with a soldier who was billeting with her and her seventeen-year-old daughter. She was angry not because the soldier got both her and her daughter pregnant and then disappeared but because, as the soldier left, he stole the mother's bicycle. "I insist on immediate return of my bicycle." Dumbfounded after meeting with the woman, Ren uncharacteristically elected not to record what advice he offered the colonel on the matter.

In contrast to the 102nd's normal activity, Ren's extracurricular adventures in England eclipsed anything stateside. He wasted no time. Fortified by George Macaulay Trevelyan's classic *A Shortened History of England* and a developing friendship with 102nd physician Lawrence Dickey, a devotee of English medical history who "actually reads" (and the surgeon who saved Vasco Hale's life), Ren used Saturdays and visiting chaplain assignments to inspect many of England's greatest historic sights. If at first he traveled by train, by late May he was joyously in possession of "the chaplain's [personal] Jeep and trailer." Immediately christened *Alabama* by Roland Rhynus—though someone's earlier name for the vehicle, *Ginger,* was left for posterity on the left rear fender—the Jeep launched Ren and friends into regular road trips. Oxford, Cambridge, Eton, Parliament, the Tower, Buckingham Palace, Westminster Abbey, and other iconic points of London—places he had long read about—he now visited. Still, as he exuded to the diary, Shakespeare territory captivated him the most:

> May 12, 1944. One of the greatest days of my life . . . [at] Stratford-on-Avon. . . . I visit Shakespeare's house where he was born. Holy Trinity Church where he is buried. Thomas Nash House . . . where he died and where he wrote "The Tempest"—The flower garden . . . every flower mentioned in the plays! I walk to Anne Hathaway's cottage. I see four figures of Hamlet, Prince Hal, Lady Macbeth and Falstaff . . . bronze . . . I go to Memorial Theater and see "Taming of the Shrew.". . . I buy some books on Shakespeare. See record of his birth at parish chapel!

As he traveled Ren repeatedly sought contact with friends and family. While one of his physician brothers, Leon, was in the Pacific theater and another, William, in Italy, his brother-in-law from Camden, Sam McNeill—like Ren too old to be drafted but still a volunteer—was "based somewhere in our area" in England with an armored division. Swamped with similar requests for contact information, both the army and the Red Cross could not help him. His searches out of Southport were fruitless. Yet at pubs, small crossroads where he asked for directions, walking around historic grounds, or just in Southport guest-preaching or watching cricket ("a very good game"), he encountered untold "average people of England" with whom he immediately engaged. Given the notable exception of a certain pregnant woman who wanted her bicycle, they were "polite," "mannered," "intelligent," "delightful," if "more reserved than [people] in the U.S." Much the opposite of these "mannered Englishmen" was another person Ren found not far from Southport: the US Army's George C. Patton. Recently relieved of command for slapping a soldier in an evacuation hospital in Italy, in late May 1944 Patton received secret orders to "command" a fake buildup of Allied forces in England to make German intelligence believe he would soon direct an invasion across the English Channel at Calais. On the morning of Monday, May 29, this diversionary assignment brought Patton to Kuntsford—forty miles inland from Southport—for a speech to civilians and another to some one thousand US Army officers trucked in from various bases. Although the Allied command found Patton's remarks that day strategically "just crazy" for his slights to the key ally, Russia, Chaplain Kennedy had a more human critique. That night he wrote Mary a terse appraisal that got by the army censors: "I will wait until I get out of the Army before expressing my feelings about the main address." Then he confided to his diary, "Lt. Gen'l Patton (Old Blood and Guts) very profane and vulgar." Still intense about the Patton experience and no doubt bridling under the censor, however, sometime after midnight he wrote Mary again and the following morning slipped it into approved mail by "helping" Warrant Officer Schmittdiel with the censoring activity. He detested Patton:

> Lt. Gen. Patton ... talks 20 minutes ... Against fox holes and slit trenches.... Man must stick to his duty and not worry about getting killed.... Your first duty is not to come out of the war alive.... Such tripe.... In every sentence profanity, blasphemy, vulgarity, obscenity.... Told medical officers to repair the slightly wounded and get them back to killing Germans—give them precedence over the desperately wounded who can never fight again.... Be fighters instead of going home and never doing anything but shovel s—. Last words of speech, "Let the fighters do the f———."... Most officers I talked with were disgusted with Patton's speech—The Leader.

Still, Ren's opinion of Patton evolved with his own actual war experience, and that approached fast. At 8:00 AM, June 6, 1944, he happened to be in the officers' club when he first learned from a German (English-language) radio broadcast of the Allied disembarkment in Normandy. With a gathering crowd he remained there for General Eisenhower's 9:30 AM announcement. In support of this long-anticipated invasion, he held a prayer service at 1:00 PM in the outside park at the Botanical Gardens. Despite a temperature of 42 degrees and "a wild wind blowing [with] a mist" and many of the unit out traveling somewhere, two hundred "Catholics, Protestants, Jews" showed up—close to half of the unit—"the largest crowd of 102nd personnel I had ever talked to at a religious service." Then it was back to the club's radio for the afternoon before heading "home" for more radio with Raymond Garton.

Some four thousand miles across the Atlantic in Camden, while spending the day by the radio, Mary wrote Ren with her Presbyterian best: "I read the Twenty-third Psalm—our Psalm you used to call it . . . [and] someone is reading the 46th Psalm over the radio." She also let him know that his Camden church resonated with approval of this dramatic development in US policy: "Your daughter [Mary Conway] rang your church bell until her hands were blistered." Likewise, just before closing his blackout curtains Ren completed a letter to Mary. It had a different tone. After summarizing the day's events in Southport and noting that his brother-in-law, Sam, was likely in the middle of the fighting in Normandy, he expressed frustration. " It . . . does not look like we are going anywhere right away. I don't want to get left out of what is going on in this invasion." Woojie the censor mailed it for him.

The army's radio news of Omaha, Utah, and the other Normandy beaches and the incursions inland—which understated the US losses—only whetted Ren's appetite. On June 26 two 102nd physicians, Thomas King and Ross King, sent over for D-day and several weeks following, returned to Southport with harrowing stories. Ren tried to stay calm as he oriented two Red Cross workers, Flora Jane Bromley and Elsie Allen, who were scheduled to travel with the 102nd and visited Southport pubs to mediate fistfights as pilots of the Royal Air Force razed the members of the 102nd for "not being fighters, just medics." With still no sign of an alert for the 102nd, on June 30 he wrangled a place in the back of a truck on a supply run, which permitted him a half day back in Stratford-on-Avon, only to return that evening to this uplifting bulletin: "Lockers to be stored in Liverpool . . . bed rolls [need to be] ready to go." With this alert going nowhere, however, his frustration returned: "I want to be in what is going on . . . that is what we came over here for." On July 4 the 102nd received another standby alert followed by a departure dance on July 5 for officers in the majestic ballroom of the Queens Hotel, overlooking Southport's promenade along the Irish Sea. Here, nurse Amy Erickson "[taught] me to dance." The next day he mailed an antique teapot to Mary and cameo rings to the girls and had a "good-bye conversation" with the Gartons in front of the fire. "They have been so good to me . . . it is like leaving home."

On July 8 another "embarrassing" postponement occurred. "The men's frustration" escalated to "drunken fights" with MPs at the Southport Botanical Gardens, requiring Ren's sociological voice of calm. At last, however, on the morning of July 14 the 102nd Evacuation Hospital marched down Lord Street, boarded a train, and headed east across England. One boxcar contained a carefully secured Jeep named *Alabama* and its canvas-covered trailer packed tight with portable altar, field communion kit, and Remington typewriter plus a case of scotch for the CO, another of bourbon for " Dan and friends," and a case of Guinness stout "not sure for who." That afternoon the 102's personnel arrived at the British army's Camp Tidworth near Southampton, looking east to the English Channel and on to France. *Alabama,* along with the rest of the unit's eighty thousand pounds of equipment, tents, supplies, and vehicles, went directly to a freighter at Southampton, then departed to await its personnel across the channel. The next day, Sunday, July 15, Ren held an outdoor service at Camp Tidworth. Having titled his sermon "Lessons of World War I," this overtly patriotic preacher nevertheless explained how a lack of Christian humility in America, France, and England had produced a haughty Treaty of Versailles—a botched peace that had ultimately led to the rise of Nazi fascism and the war they now had to go fight. He hoped that, when World War II ended, such mistakes of hubris could be avoided. That evening he pondered whether "any" in front of him that morning had digested what he said. Conclusion: "Unlikely." He then went out into a night punctuated with exploding German buzz bombs to meet Dan Laws and Joe Rutenberg for "sledge-hammers"—shots of vodka and lime juice. Before heading to bed "mildly sedated" he told the diary that, while "nervous," he found everything "very interesting" in "Buzztown."

PART TWO

France

As I said before, throughout much of the fall of 2007 we stayed pretty close to home in Pennedepie and Honfleur. Granted, there was a Friday night in Paris to see Marc and Béatrice's son, Sebastian, in a musical review at the old Trianon theater (followed by a four-course dinner at the family's Paris home that *started* at 12:30 AM), as well as three different runs to the D-day sites. Still, as that winter came on, I was deep in the work with late-afternoon explorations of Upper Normandy, especially the array of German bunkers still lining the English Channel. And that was when my light bulb finally came on. Through the current reality of the war around us I began to see that the French countryside and its people might yield far more detail than just the route followed by the 102nd and the different locations where it operated. By late November, with the substantial aid of Marc's cousin, Christine Bouchon, Susan and I were negotiating every twist and turn of the 102nd as it moved throughout Lower Normandy and Brittany. And we turned up a lot—key unmarked sites and even more endearing people with splendid memories. By December 2007, with a rented diesel Peugeot that got fifty-two clean-burning miles per gallon on the highway—increasingly appreciated as fuel pushed the equivalent of $8.50 a US gallon—we were knocking on doors that eventually led us to some of the most poignant moments in the life of the 102nd. But let the chaplain guide us there.

The Overseas World of the 102nd Evacuation Hospital

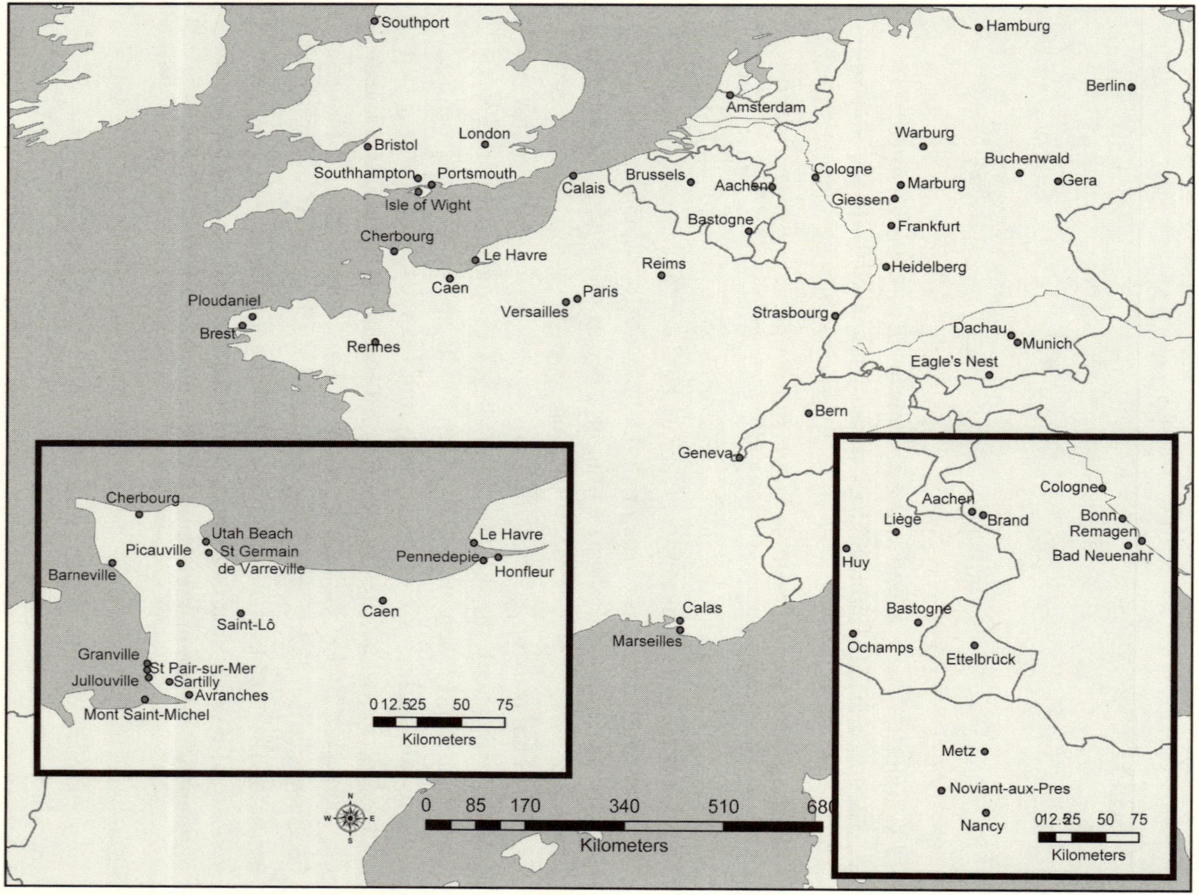

A map of southern England, France, and western Germany, with detail insets of places crucial in *The Chaplain's Conflict*. Cartography by Steve Padgett-Vasquez.

CHAPTER 4

Utah Beach

July 18–19, 1944

At 4:30 PM on Monday, July 17, 1944, personnel of the 102nd Evacuation Hospital boarded the sixteen-hundred-ton *Laird's Isle,* formerly a private English excursion steamer that had been transporting Allied troops across the English Channel ever since D-day, June 6. While waiting for a full convoy to assemble, *Laird's Isle* moved down the channel and anchored for the night off the Isle of Wight. Ren went "to bed in [a] hammock . . . [after an] interesting day . . . [seeing the] beautiful coast of Isle of Wight" even though "the protective barrage balloon drifting lazily overhead brought the thought of war very close indeed." At 4:00 PM the next afternoon the ten-vessel convoy followed a minesweeper across the channel to Cherbourg, then headed northeast, where *Laird's Isle* peeled to anchor at 6:00 PM a mile off Omaha Beach "in a park of 100 ships." After staring at the "steep bank at Omaha," where "thousands died [on] D-Day," Ren and the 102nd boarded LCS (landing craft support) vessels and ran west fifteen miles to disembark at Utah Beach.

Ren's LCT (landing craft, tank) beached in the long and silvery light of a July evening at latitude forty-nine, where darkness comes at 11:00 PM. "I step on shore . . . at 8:15 PM, July 18, 1944. I carry my duffle bag, weighs 100 lbs, my musette bag, gas mask, pistol *belt,* plus canteen and trench coat and bag of rations . . . carry all this off pier . . . 150 yds along shore and another 150 yds up over sand dune . . . almost exhausted. Woojie . . . comes out to help me last 25 yds but I did not need him." While waiting an hour for the 102nd to unload "Rutenberg, Poirer and I . . . go over to wire pens to see German prisoners there right by landing pier, an unhappy scene for them." One POW, apparently worried about what would happen next, recognized the chaplain's cross on Ren's field jacket. In English he asked, "Father, can you give me Last Rites?" "I am Protestant," Ren replied, "but I can pray with you for a moment if you want." They did.

By July 18 more than one million Allied forces had pushed through much of Germany's Atlantic Wall. In addition, US soldiers had liberated the Cotentin Peninsula, including highly fortified Cherbourg, and British forces had freed Caen, thereby moving the offensive toward Paris. Over a month of brutal fighting remained in the interior of France, however. As Ren trudged across Utah's dunes, just thirty miles inland US forces to the southeast concluded the bloody battle for Saint-Lô. To support this action and the general push into Brittany, Commanding Officer Goodiel had orders to organize the operations of the 102nd forty miles across the peninsula, near Barneville-le-Carteret. At this port, liberated on June 18, their equipment awaited them. Now they were part of the Third Army. And now—returned to a real command—George C. Patton was their general though Ren would never set eyes on the "vulgar" one again.

To get to Barneville they left the beach that night at 9:30 PM. Remember, at that latitude in that month, darkness comes late. They marched an hour and a half inland—some six miles—down a dusty road and over sand dunes to expansive pastures one hundred yards from tiny Saint-Germain-de-Varreville, right where the US 4th Infantry had paused on D-day. There, along with one thousand other troops, including the 39th Evac, they fell asleep on the ground, Ren wrapped in field jacket and a "fine" Burberry trench coat under him and poncho on top. As he lay down he was worried about the fast pace that Executive Officer Sutherland had set for the march, not too difficult for officers carrying light packs but tough on "the men" with "full packs," plus the officers' other gear, as well as two ward tents. ("I asked First Sgt. if he wants break for men; he says let it go.") Exhaustion quickly offset these thoughts. He slept. Such concerns, however, were still with him the next morning when he bounced up at 7:00 AM, ready for World War II. Fortified less by a cold shave "out of helmet" and more by "very good" heated breakfast of C-ration stew, Ren "had a long talk with the Col. about . . . hard march," not that hard on "officers and nurses" but unnecessarily difficult for "the men." Goodiel gave "little response."

CHAPTER 5

Barneville-le-Carteret and Picauville

JULY 1944

At 8:15 PM on July 19, the 102nd departed Saint-Germaine-de-Varreville in trucks moving southeast across the Cotentin—"blasted towns" everywhere. At 11:15 PM they set up in another pasture two miles north of Barneville. As promised, all of the unit's equipment awaited them—including *Alabama,* with booze unbroken—personnel tents even erected. With still-fresh memories of Goffs, Ren returned to sleeping on a bedroll and cot in a pyramidal tent shared with buddies Laws, King, Peterson, and Rutenberg. The next day he awoke to find that Goodiel had added to his list of chaplain's duties the locating of laundry services for the physicians; the 102nd's washing machine serviced hospital sheets and occasionally "men's laundry." Bemused yet excited about any excuse to explore, off he went in *Alabama* with the dirty clothes of at least eight physicians—first stop seven miles inland to the north at Surtainville. He located a woman who had directed an elementary school at nearby Valognes until it was blown up a month earlier. She spoke "a little English" and was eager for the take-in work. Here he also had the first of many encounters with Europe's "other" wartime rural economy. "Small boy . . . tries to sell me a 4 oz bottle of cognac for 200 francs." As he drove back to Barneville, however, his bemusement about the laundry assignment gave way to more pondering about "the men" unnecessarily struggling over the Utah dunes two days before. Finding the CO this time willing to go along with anything, back at the tents "I speak to 75 officers and nurses about their treatment of the men . . . flunkies . . . [making them] carry their duffle bags, etc. I offended some."

The next morning these concerns again moved to the back burner. Overnight Goodiel received new orders. Up at 4:30 AM and with some of the officers' laundry left at Surtainville, the 102nd trucked back across the Cotentin twenty-two miles east to become fully operational out of a pasture at Picauville, across the road from a P47 airbase, between Pont-l'Abbé and Sainte-Mère-Église, where the 101st Airborne had torturously helped begin D-day operations back on the night of June 5. Even if German planes could target the hospital, it was still relatively safe while being close enough—between ten and twenty miles away—to recovery from the Saint-Lô battle and westerly fighting at Periers and Lessay. Little action occurred that first day in Picauville; Ren and Roland even got orders to take *Alabama* the twenty miles back to Surtainville to pick up and drop off more laundry.

On July 21, however, the wounded started arriving. For the week following that date, the hospital stayed 50 percent full, averaging two hundred patients a day. The load was made more demanding by rapid arrivals of seven or more wounded at a time, all needing instant surgery. The 102nd moved to a combat schedule of twelve hours on and twelve hours off. Indeed, just four days into France, the surgeons had to expand into the command's pyramidal tent, which moved offices, including Ren's, into pup tents. As Ren told the diary on the night of July 25, "the 102nd is [now] in the war." And the next night he continued to Mary:

> Ambulance after ambulance came . . . the flood . . . surgeons working day and night (there are two shifts) . . . and the boys . . . exhausted when they come in from lack of sleep and pain . . . don't have much to say and are very patient and brave . . . It was so bloody. One man with shrapnel [was] William Gregory from Selma, lives out on the Summerfield Road.

Ren's chaplain duties during this week went on "practically all day" in the wards. "Some boys want a prayer . . . one wanted to take Communion [so] I took some wine in a paper cup and a piece of bread in my hand and gave it to him." But Ren had secular issues, too. Consistent with the Geneva Convention, the US Army's ambulances picked up wounded German POWs as they brought in GIs, and some twenty of these received treatment under the tents at Picauville. "A few of the [GIs] in the wards give [the German soldiers] cigarettes" because most were conscripted Poles known to hate Germany and to "shoot duds" at the GIs whenever possible. Others wanted them "out," however, and throughout the week Ren had mediation talks with the intensely disagreeing GI patients. Ultimately, when "one GI [patient] said he was going to kill" the POWs, Ren read the tensions as unnecessary, along with everything else going on, and recommended that the POWs be segregated in a separate tent. They moved to "one ward—D-4." For the chaplain there was also the role of medical social worker.

With battle coming to an end, after four deaths in the hospital (one a German sniper) and more than two hundred patients evacuated back to England out of the P47 airstrip across the road, life in the 102nd eased up on July 26. That afternoon Ren and Roland made a laundry pickup at Surtainville. A few miles into their return, at a tiny intersection they encountered none other than Ren's brother-in-law from Camden, Sam McNeill, on a short break from tough fighting at the nearby front as a gunner and driver on one of Patton's half-tracks. Thrilled to offer *Alabama*'s rolling hospitality, Ren took Sam "in my Jeep" on a tour of Picauville and the 102nd, then returned him to his buddies, who had been conveniently delayed by cognac in Surtainville.

"Freed cognac" also flowed in Picauville. On Sunday night, July 30, although Ren sought that morning to calm the waters with a brief sermon on "Why We Are Here," cognac laced with medical alcohol from the pathology/mortuary tents commanded more attention among the surgeons and nurses. That night three physicians "got drunk in our hospital in the presence of patients ... cussing, loud, noisy ... disgusting performance before patients." Physician Ed Peterson, although no saint, stayed deeply concerned about that night; for years after the war he remembered the drinking as "beyond anything I ever saw on the *M*A*S*H* television show." Ren always viewed such extreme drinking much as he viewed General Patton's vocabulary—"vulgar" and essentially unnecessary for winning the war. Still, the chaplain himself was not that far away from regular, if generally disciplined, indulgence in medical alcohol as the regular stress reliever in an evacuation hospital.

At midday on August 1 Goodiel headed his unit west toward Granville, which had been liberated with little fighting the day before, to deal with mounting casualties from Patton's push for the "breakthrough" at Avranches and also the developing battle for Saint-Malo. Whether it was "fog" from medical alcohol or confusion due just to the chaos of war, Goodiel gave the wrong map coordinates to the lead vehicles. By 9:00 PM the 102nd had finally progressed twenty miles to the point of bivouac, a pasture just outside of Buisson and two miles south of Lessay, where battle had raged five days earlier. The next morning, while Goodiel awaited radio orders as to what precise location near Granville he should head toward, Ren's exploration of neighboring Château Blanc in Buisson was cut short when he encountered a few of the "men" from the 102nd "looting" a home and "the owner runs them out." Now, MP duties for the chaplain. Finally at 2:00 AM the next morning, August 1, Goodiel had the 102nd under way again. By 7:30 AM the lead vehicles had reached the target spot of pastures just outside the hamlet of Saint-Pair-sur-Mer, five miles west of Granville and ten miles short of Avranches, where the fighting had climaxed only twenty-four hours earlier. "Most of the convoy" got lost, however, and with "many of the men drunk . . . 15 of them dead drunk," the bulk of the 102nd rolled in around noon. Ren's diary distilled it this way: "A snafu day—worst I have seen in the 102nd."

CHAPTER 6

Saint-Pair-sur-Mer

August 1944

Before I can tell you what happened to Ren and his friends in and around Saint-Pair-sur-Mer, I need to tell you what happened to Susan and me there. Here, in the poignant confluence of two stories—the 102nd's and that of local French civilians—we bore down on a seminal moment in the chaplain's war: when he gave a Bible to a dead girl.

After a half day of using Ren's notes to try to locate the precise spot where the 102nd had set up—but failing—we paid a cold call on the only official we could find in a ten-mile radius, the irrepressible seventy-four-year-old Louis Forget, mayor of the neighboring town of Jullouville. He spoke some English, and he knew all about "the American hospital." It had been located adjacent to his father's farm. However, he was up for reelection and had a full afternoon of appointments. Could we come back? Did we want him to line up conversations with others who remembered the 102nd? For sure. On the way out we asked whether he knew the Garnier family—the family of a girl named Bleuette Garnier, whose death at the age of twelve, under a tent of the 102nd, deeply touched our Protestant chaplain. In her memory Ren gave the child's parents an English Bible. I wanted to send a photograph of the Bible to Ren's daughter, Mary Conway, who had been extraordinarily helpful in the whole project. Louis did not know the Garnier family, but he said he would ask around.

A month later we were back at Louis's office. Although he had struck out on finding any Garnier family members still living in the area, he had a day of appointments set up for us. None of these people spoke English, he explained, and the conversations would be more complicated than we could handle in our "nonnative tongue." "We will be talking about many horrible deaths." He spent the day by our side.

We first visited with seventy-nine-year-old Jean Touzé, owner of the Angomesnil camping park. He recalled that, as a child, he had watched a movie at the hospital; the "commander" had let him in the tent, where he sat alongside doctors and nurses. One doctor belched a lot. Even if he did not recall the name of the movie, Jean certainly remembered the makeup of the hospital, for he had lived just across the road from it. He presented us with a detailed map of the tents—reflecting a logical adjustment of the "ideal" configuration as detailed in the army's *Medical Field Manual,* which based the layout on local features, such as the Thar River. The explorations of young Jean were resurrected in expertly color-coded cartography, down to where the bodies of the soldiers who had just died were kept—the same tent where the personnel stored the alcohol they drank.

Next we met Madame Roland Dulins Duprey, who had lost two brothers to accidents involving leftover German grenades. Although she had no recollections of a Garnier family, she had a childhood friend, Marie Louise Lévi-Ménard, who "remembered everyone." Off we went to find Madame Lévi-Ménard in the modern hospital in nearby Granville, where she was recovering from knee surgery. She was seventy-nine but looked fifty-five. Striking. No, she knew of no Bleuette Garnier, but there in the hospital room—where Pennie of Pennedepie finally found the limits of French tolerance for dogs—Madame Lévi-Ménard recounted her life as an eighteen-year-old member of the Resistance.

Her family had rented the manse that once was used by the priests of Saint-Aubin-des-Préaux, adjacent to Saint-Pair-sur-Mer. When the Germans took control of the area, the officers set up shop in the downstairs of the manse, while the family moved upstairs. Despite their late-night presence below, Marie Louise used her professional skills as a shorthand transcriber, combined with a battery-powered radio receiver made by her cousin, an electrician, in order to record forbidden BBC broadcasts on the Allied troop movements. The following mornings her transcriptions were passed on to a local Resistance network. Indeed, a week before D-day she augmented her arsenal by stealing a typewriter from a stack of German supplies—a theft facilitated by the lack of electric lights in many small towns of Normandy that had resulted when the Germans confiscated the coal that otherwise would have fueled the power plants. During daylight hours she hid the typewriter under Saint-Aubin's confessional booth across the street, where she had also been keeping her radio equipment. Suffice it to say that, by the time the *débarquement* started on June 6, her Resistance friends were getting neatly typed transcriptions of the unfolding liberation, possibly better intelligence than the "house guests" had.

Marie Louise kept talking, hardly skipping a beat (though frowning)

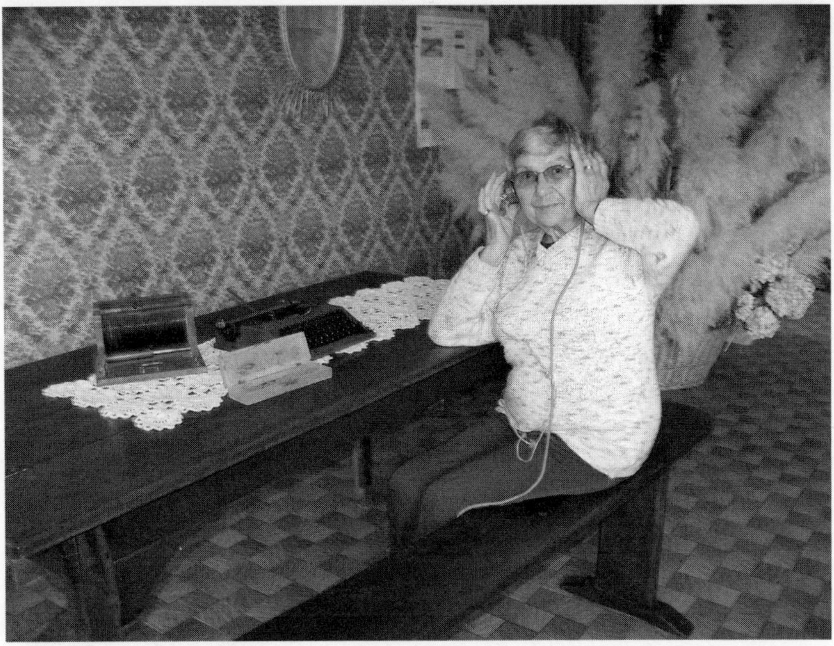

Marie Louise Lévi-Ménard in her Bréville-sur-Mer home, demonstrating the stolen German typewriter and homemade radio receiver she used to transcribe forbidden BBC battle news in German-occupied Saint-Aubin-des-Préaux, France (October 2010). Photo by Susan McWilliams.

when a large nurse evacuated Pennie to an adjacent patio. She explained how she had moved to Paris after the war to look for work and wound up marrying a Jewish gentleman who had escaped the concentration camps because, as a French soldier, he was considered a POW. Together they had built a highly successful clothing business, which they sold in 1980 to retire in Normandy. She then returned to the origin of our conversation. Numerous French children met accidental deaths after the Allies arrived. The name "Bleuette," however, was not familiar to her. Perhaps on some future visit we should talk with her friend Marie-Thérèse. In fact, three weeks later she was scheduled to return to her château, which faced the Bay of Mont-Saint-Michel, and she asked us to come for an overnight visit. We would be able to see her radio, her transcripts, and her photographs of restored US Army trucks and Jeeps used in current D-day celebrations all over Lower Normandy. Susan inquired about our bringing Pennie. "Mais oui, madame."

Two weeks later, with Madame Lévi-Ménard still in the hospital, we were back at Louis's office. He had arranged a full day. During the last visit

Madame Duprey offered the same suggestion that Madame Lévi-Ménard had: For a Bleuette Garnier, check with Marie-Thérèse Desroches. She had been "injured" when the 102nd was in the area and might have helpful recollections. Louis now had her lined up. At age seventy-four Madame Desroches indeed still had vivid memories. With all of us seated at her dining room table she began by telling us her maiden name—Provost. I felt a rush of adrenalin; Ren had noted that a Provost family was in the hospital that fateful night. She continued. She and others were walking home from church. Her brother picked up a grenade left along the road by the fleeing Germans. It exploded. Reluctantly she showed us the scars on her left arm. Susan then asked if others were hurt as well. "Yes, several hurt and one killed—Bleuette died." Despite being a large man with an artificial knee and heart problems, Louis still has a few of the quick moves he had needed as a French officer in Algeria in the 1960s. As he jumped up out of that chair, with eyes flicking back and forth between Susan and me, he muttered, "Did you say Bleuette? Did you say Bleuette Garnier?" "Non monsieur, Bleuette Bindel." The Bindels had apparently been gone from the area "forever." And who knows? Could there have been two Bleuettes? Or could Ren have written the wrong last name? Not like him to do that. We pressed, but there was little more.

A month later, at Louis's email urging, we were back. He had found what Madame Desroches had predicted. No Bindels. However, on a hunch he went poking around the graveyard in nearby Sartilly, where Madame Desroches had been injured. There he found a gravestone for a Bleuette Bindel. That morning we met Madame Desroches at Sartilly. We saw the gravestone, which had a touching photograph embedded on the front—Bleuette in her first-Communion dress. However, more important was the death date, which matched what Ren had written in the diary: "6 August 1944." Madame Desroches walked us to the spot where the explosion had occurred and recounted the tragic details. We had found Bleuette. According to the diary, a Garnier family also had children in the hospital on the night of August 6, and in the chaos Ren confused the two. Here was major progress. Still, as for the Bindels and the Bible Ren had given them . . . we drove back to Pennedepie fresh out of leads.

Three weeks passed, and the mail brought a kind note from Madame Lévi-Ménard. When were we coming for the overnight visit? Susan and I had been envisioning the possibilities of some social life between Louis and Marie Louise inasmuch as both had deceased spouses. So back we went with luncheon reservations for five (including Pennie), to be followed by an afternoon and evening with Marie Louise's memorabilia. To our knowledge no French romance surfaced on that visit, but something else did. The next morning on our way home we took a slight detour through Sartilly. When nothing else remains, knock on doors and say "Bonjour." By this time Susan's French was really good. She asked the fiftyish woman at the front desk in the mayor's office in Sartilly whether she knew anything about Bleuette Bindel's gravestone down the road. "Why don't you ask Bleuette's sister?" came the reply. "She is married; her name is Dominique Lucas, and she lives in Saint-Martin-des-Champs, about forty miles from here. We went to school together." "Mais, oui, madame!" You see, after Bleuette died, her parents—like many other families shattered by war—tried to escape their pain by having additional children (in the Bindels' case, eight more). Indeed, as late as 1953 they welcomed infant Dominique Bindel.

Two weeks later we arrived at the home of Dominique Lucas in Saint-Martin-des-Champs. Dominique had not only extensive family photographs but also Bleuette's report cards and a school essay in which she wrote in perfect script, "I want to grow up to be a good person. I want my mother and father to be proud of me." In turn, Dominique connected us with another sister, Yvette, age eighty-two, married and living at Caen, not far from Pennedepie—and who had been there for it all on August 6, 1944: the explosion, followed by Bleuette's death. In the end Susan and I never found Ren's Bible—really, Bleuette's Bible.

But here is what we *did* find.

Despite its ignominious entrance into Saint-Pair-sur-Mer on August 1, 1944, by nightfall the unit was fully functional and about as "semipermanent" as possible without being housed in buildings. Spread across four acres of pasture adjacent to the Thar River and facing route D21 were thirty-five tents for hospital wards, personnel, administration, mess (one for enlisted men, another for officers), and a Red Cross tent, which doubled as a chapel—as well as a motor pool and an ambulance parking lot. With diesel-powered generators the large washing machine and two drinking-water filters churned with water from the Thar. One mile east and next to Bouillon a landing strip with wire tarmac overlooked the prewar resort of Jullouville, whose majestic beaches fronted the English Channel. Two days earlier fighter planes had departed from this tarmac to strafe German installations at Avranches. The strip now hosted planes evacuating patients from the 102nd and also from the Red Cross hos-

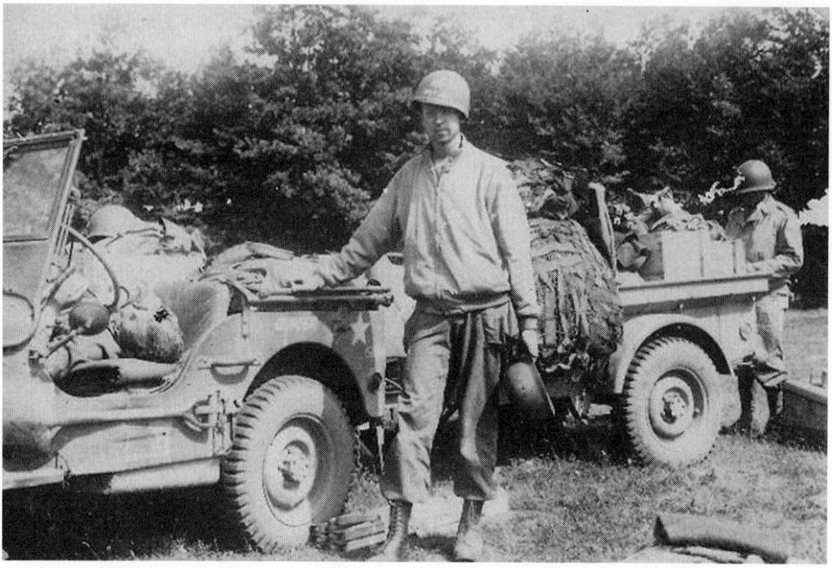

Pfc. Roland Rhynus (left) and RCK just before unloading *Alabama* and trailer (with chaplain's gear and booze) at the 102nd's camp near Saint-Pair-sur-Mer, France (August 1944). Note original name of Jeep, *Ginger,* on left rear fender. Unknown photographer. RCK Papers.

pital in the Jullouville casino, which had been a German hospital until July 26. Indeed, at this stop the 102nd barely missed Eisenhower himself. In late August, just as the 102nd moved on, the Supreme Headquarters Allied Expeditionary Force moved into a Jullouville school complex—La Colonie Scolaire de Saint-Ouen—and General Eisenhower took up residence at one of the striking châteaux on D911, overlooking the Bay of Mont-Saint-Michel, just seven miles from the 102nd's campsite. Ren's new home.

The first two weeks at Saint-Pair revealed a larger version of the hospital life the 102nd had experienced at Picauville. Since much of the ground fighting occurred during the day and some four hours might be needed to move a casualty from the front to a field hospital and then back to the 102nd, ambulances normally began arriving at the 102nd in early afternoon and continued until dawn the next day. Two days into full operation, on August 4, at 1:00 PM eighty beds were filled; by midnight 200 were filled (out of a standard maximum of 400), and seventy patients were waiting in the shock ward. By the following morning, after evacuation runs to the Bouillon airstrip, 225 beds had patients. Five days later, however, all 300 beds were full even after evacuations.

The staccato rhythm of the hospital easily permitted Ren to keep *Alabama* moving in the community with the officers' laundry and to offer morning services in the Red Cross tent on both Sunday, August 6, and Sunday, August 13. Still, his chief chaplain duties remained in the wards, saying prayers, giving Communion, and just talking with the GIs. Around 20 percent of the patients were German POWs, now segregated, and the language barrier continually frustrated Ren. ("I do not speak any German!") With an expanding repertoire of French "words and phrases" he did a little better with the local civilians who were brought to "l'hôpital militaire américain." French children in particular connected with the personnel of the 102nd. Jean Touzé, age sixteen, marveled at his first sight of a washing machine and, along with several friends, watched 16 mm movies outdoors at the 102nd as guests of Lieutenant Colonel Sutherland. Likewise, young Louis Forget traded his father's "borrowed" calvados for packs of cocoa powder and his first driving lesson in a Jeep, which he sublimely drove into a stone barn near the airstrip. "My legs were too short to reach the pedals effectively." *Alabama* sustained no serious damage.

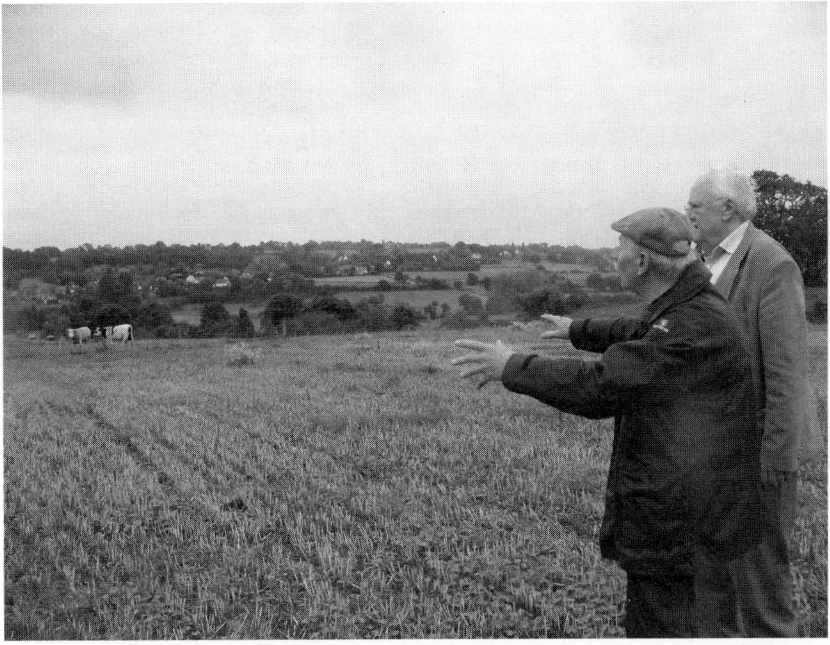

Jean Touzé (left) and Louis Forget at the pasture along the Thar River, reliving what Touzé had drawn in his detailed diagram of the 102nd's camp near Saint-Pair-sur-Mer, France (October 2010). Photo by Susan McWilliams.

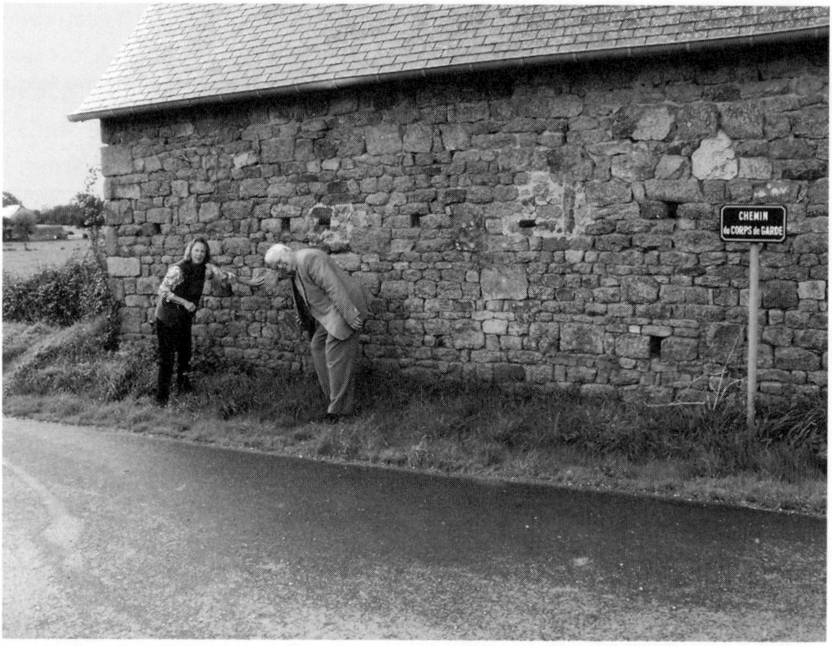

The author's wife, Susan, and Mayor Louis Forget feel the indentions in the side of the stone barn where youthful Louis, in August 1944, crashed a US Army jeep (October 2010). Photo by the author.

More poignant is the manner in which its medical expertise profoundly connected the 102nd with the locals. Accidentally run over by a US Army truck, Ferdinand Periers died only after the surgeons tried for "hours" to treat his severe head injuries. Less tragic, other children—perhaps three—who were hit by army vehicles walked away from the hospital with appropriate casts and bandages, as did the adult who was shot in the arm by a drunk GI. None of these civilian casualties captured Ren's intensity more, however, than the children who were hurt while playing with the multitude of live grenades discarded or lost by German troops who had so recently fled the area. While off-target American bombs involved in the fighting at Saint-Lô and Avranches apparently killed more children than German grenades around Saint-Pair-sur-Mer, "at least five children" became accidental grenade victims during the two weeks the 102nd worked in the area. These young casualties included the Dulins brothers—Rémy, age seven, who died instantly, and Michel, age twelve, who died in surgery at the 102nd.

Ren was observing such surgeries the evening of Sunday, August 6, when an army ambulance brought in others hurt in a grenade explosion two miles west in Sartilly. Lucienne Provost was walking home from services at l'église de Sartilly with her children, Marie-Thérèse, age eleven, and Maurice, age nine, and a friend's daughters, Bleuette Bindel, age twelve, and Yvette Bindel, seven. As they approached the intersection of routes D35 and D335 in front of the cemetery, Maurice spotted a grenade in the bushes on the right side of the road. He picked it up. His mother immediately shouted, "Put that down! I have told you not to play with grenades." Maurice dropped the grenade. It exploded. While some of the random shrapnel hit Marie-Thérèse's left arm, most of it flew into Bleuette's upper body and head.

A 102nd ambulance happened by within five minutes of the explosion and brought the four children and Madame Provost to the 102nd tents, her husband arriving shortly thereafter with Bleuette's parents. It was a typical intense evening: surgery full, wounded GIs waiting in the shock ward, three hundred patients in recovery and elsewhere. Fifteen of

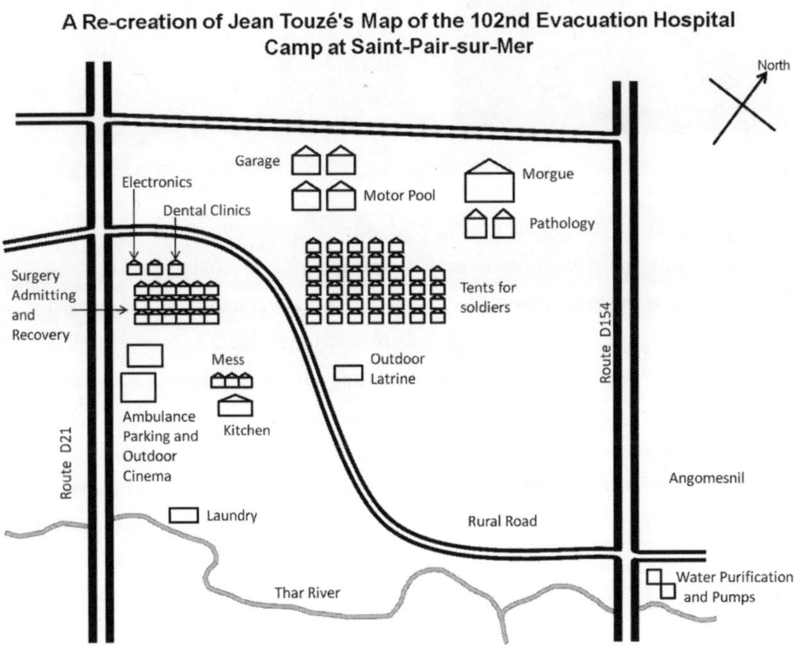

Schematic showing the setup of the 102nd Evacuation Hospital near Saint-Pair-sur-Mer, France, based on original sketch by Jean Touzé. Cartography by Steve Padgett-Vasquez.

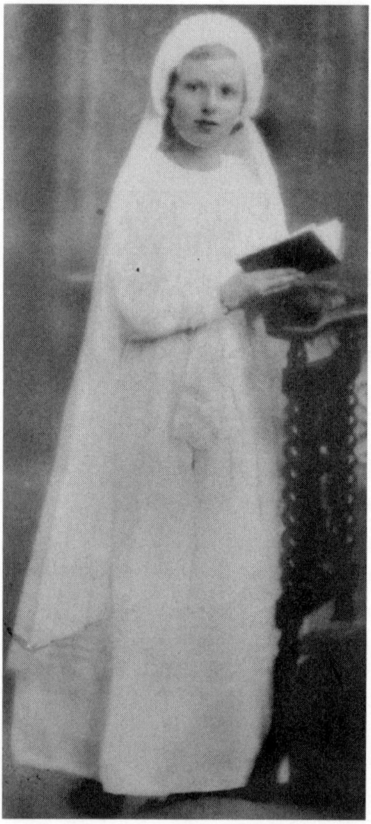

Bleuette Bindel at First Communion, Sartilly, France (1943). Unknown photographer. Photo courtesy of Yvette Bindel.

the injured were French civilians, and one of them was Bleuette's friend René Garnier, age ten. Those in the ambulance found Maurice, Yvette, and Madame Provost physically unhurt. Then, because of the backlog of patients, they transported Marie-Thérèse to the Red Cross Hospital in Jullouville for treatment of her lacerations, which left deep, striated scars that would remain forever on her lower left arm.

They moved Bleuette immediately back to surgery, where the surgeons worked on her for some four hours. During that time Ren sat on a cot in the admitting tent with Bleuette's parents, Louis and Louise Bindel—both longtime postal workers. The poignancy of it all intensified because "I could not talk French with them much," and his ineffective efforts at translating a few passages from a New Testament were made even more difficult by the war outside: "Jerries [were] overhead . . . heavy bombing . . . got ammunition dump near here." Bleuette died that night on the operating table. Ren softly ushered the Bindels, cradling Bleuette's body, to a waiting ambulance. He had nothing else he could give, so he gave them the English-language Testament he used in the tent. Sad and frustrated, he finally turned in that night, thinking about the fragility of his own daughters—Mary Conway and Margaret—and to one of his recurring sermon thoughts about evil: "To war nothing whatsoever is sacred, and anything at all may be violated."

The morning after Bleuette died, Commanding Officer Goodiel asked Ren to talk with him about the "discontent" in his "organization," which had been underscored the day before by Adjutant Basil Winstead's telling the CO that he wanted out of the 102nd. They talked from 9 AM to 11 AM about "where [Goodiel] had done wrong, where he [had] failed" as the CO. The chaplain, now acting as organizational psychologist, praised Winstead's administrative mind and agreed with Goodiel's assessment of a serious morale problem in the unit. Ren emphasized that the doctors and nurses were strong in delivering medical care and that "occasional" drunkenness might be excused due to the extreme stress. Still, the morale problems would not go away, and medical care could not get even better unless the doctors and nurses quit treating "the men" as "flunkies." The medical personnel themselves needed to be "managed" not by the misguided and "detested" authoritarianism of surgery chief William Stewart and of nursing chief Frances Ewing but by consistent and balanced leadership from the top of the unit. Goodiel said he would address these matters in the next twenty-four hours. In turn, Ren promised to talk with Winstead about remaining. Winstead agreed to stay. The CO apparently did nothing.

These last several days now flowed together. Ren's sorrow over Bleuette's death merged with collective fatigue ("little sleep for four days") and frustration—unlike any "down" since entering the army. So, undoubtedly to the detriment of his duties to the two hundred patients still in the wards, Ren received Sutherland's approval for a half day of exploring up closer to the front. On the morning of August 11 he and Roland Rhynus headed off in the Jeep westerly through Avranches and back along the coast to Saint-James to a massive, temporary cemetery for US casualties not fortunate enough to have made it to evacuation. If this was supposed to be self-designed therapy, it failed. When they arrived, "125 bodies [lay] on the grass awaiting burial . . . most from 6th Armored Div [killed at Saint-Lô and Saint-Malo] . . . bodies [placed] in mattress covers and [ready to] bury." His earlier feelings merged into a singularly overwhelming "bad" feeling. Beyond the bodies, out at sea stood the iconic sixteenth-century

Mont-Saint-Michel—one of the greatest historic sites of Europe. Ren the scholar hardly glanced at it. By 2:30 PM they were back in Saint-Pair. "I go out and lie on grass." Yet, after he had slept for six hours, his irrepressible fascination with everything around him gradually returned. By the next afternoon, Saturday, August 12, with evacuations moving swiftly and admissions way down, *Alabama* headed back to Mont-Saint-Michel. "I walk through the streets . . . climb the steps to the abbey and the church, wander around the subterranean passages through the rock—very old, quaint, beautiful, narrow, curving." Aesthetic adjectives spoke to the palliatives of a good night's sleep and a wonder in stone.

For the time being this "up" continued. While Ren was in Mont-Saint-Michel Goodiel received word that the front lines of Patton's Third Army were moving into Brittany so fast that he was to start loading the 102nd, then stand by for a new location to the west. The next day as they waited, "the French came in great numbers" to say goodbye. They "presented many flowers," and a "mayor" read a resolution of appreciation for the soldiering, as well as the doctoring. Afterward, Ren "gather[ed] up remains of our meals—K-rations—and [took] it out to the road and [gave] it to the French people," undoubtedly regretting that something equally substantive could not have been done for Bleuette's parents. For one more day the 102nd waited; Ren used the time to guide Dan Laws through Mont-Saint-Michel.

The 102nd then headed for Brittany on the afternoon of Wednesday, August 16, covering some fifty-five miles before bivouacking in another pasture just east of Dinan, where "after chow" the "Jeep's-eye" tour continued: "Dinan—a beautiful old French city." On the road again at 7 AM they covered sixty miles—Ren catching both flowers and onions pitched by the welcoming French—to spend the night in yet another pasture on the periphery of Guingamp. After another seventy miles on Friday, August 18, the 102nd pulled into its next base of operation, Ploudaniel, just ten miles east of Brest. Two truckloads of nurses were missing. They chugged in that night with extra flowers and harrowing stories about being lost and muddling through a crossroads near Lesneven, which was still occupied by straggling but well-armed German soldiers. No shots fired.

CHAPTER 7

Ploudaniel

August–September 1944

At Ploudaniel the 102nd set up its tents in broad pasture lands two hundred yards north of the sixteenth-century Château de Trébodennic. However, once again, before I can tell you what happened here, I need to tell you how Susan and I found ourselves inside this rambling place.

Ren's diary provides the precise location for Château de Trébodennic. Before making the four-hour drive southeast to find it, I checked the Internet. The château was still in the hands of the family that owned it when the 102nd came through; they leased it for weddings and other major events and welcomed inquiries by telephone and mail—no email. Susan sent a letter to Madame Anne Louboutin-Croc explaining our interests in a particular major event, World War II. Two months passed and no response. So off we went to Ploudaniel, ready to try the upbeat "Bonjour." At *centre-ville* Ploudaniel a sign pointed us to this stately artifact of ancient Brittany. Repeated knocks on the main door, however, got the same results as the letter. After a brief walk around the grounds we spotted a light in one of the outbuildings. Perhaps "Bonjour" would get its chance after all. Although the kind woman who greeted us spoke like lightning, we finally got her point. She was the resident manager, and the owner, while living in Ploudaniel—though not in the château—was away in Paris. I left a business card with our Pennedepie address on the back. In a culture where personal and professional cards assume an almost iconic role, perhaps this would help. On the way out of town a small marker on the side of a building caught Susan's eye. It honored one Aimé Talec, a Resistance leader who had been tortured and imprisoned by the Germans. Susan photographed it and we headed home.

Normal Pennedepie life ensued. No word from Ploudaniel. Three months later, as we planned another exploratory run down to Brittany, however, a letter arrived. Madame Sylvie Louboutin-Croc advised that neither she nor her daughter-in-law, Anne, were in Ploudaniel when we first visited. Could we please return? "Mais oui, madame." An exchange of letters established the plan. Three weeks hence we were to appear at Mayor Joël Marchadour's office in Ploudaniel. There would be a reception, then a meeting in the mayor's conference room, where we could talk with those folks who remembered the 102nd. From there we would adjourn to Château de Trébodennic and its pastures.

Madame Louboutin-Croc had written to us in Parisian French, so, driving into Ploudaniel, we were somewhat nervous about our ability to communicate. I took out my anxiety on Susan: "What if this is a gold mine of information about the 102nd, but we understand only half of what they say? Will everybody talk as fast as the resident manager?" Before Susan could come up with a calming response, we saw her. There at the front of the mayor's office was Madame Louboutin-Croc. With adrenalin suddenly eclipsing anxiety, I approached her primed with my best "Bonjour." Before I could get it out, however, this tiny and elegant eighty-something lady greeted me: "Hello, I'm Sylvie. Welcome to Ploudaniel." Over the next three hours and with the smoothness of a UN interpreter she translated the most complicated conversations, many about death. In the process we learned that she and her husband had spent the immediate postwar years in Paris, where, to achieve anything major in government or business, one spoke English. "You know, the Marshall Plan." We also pieced together that she had inherited the château from her husband, Pierre Louboutin-Croc, who lived there during the war with its longtime owners, his aunt and uncle, Monsieur and Madame Louis Croc, who adopted him right after the war.

That afternoon's visit to Trébodennic was only a start. Sylvie wanted us to meet her family and more of her friends. While I was hunting information on the 102nd, she wanted them to know more about the life of Captain Renwick C. Kennedy from Camden, Alabama, who had paid more than one visit to her family's grand place. So, three weeks later, it was back to the office of Mayor Joël Marchadour: an 11 AM reception with toasts to the US Army drawing on champagne, scotch, and bourbon—Jack Daniels costs more in Birmingham than it does in Ploudaniel—followed by more interviews with people Sylvie had rounded up. Then Sylvie hosted a seated luncheon for twelve in her home adjacent to the château. At eighty-three she cooked and then seamlessly served a roast of pork, marinated in champagne and the juice of blood oranges, accompanied by three different wines and two hours of conversation, more French than English. After this classic French luncheon we wound our

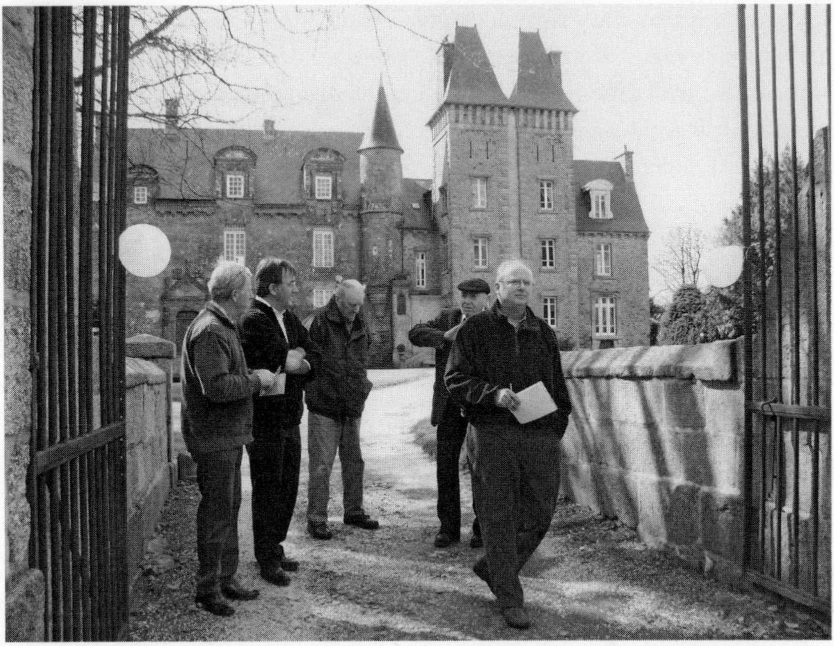

The author (with notebook) at the gates to Château de Trébodennic, with (in background, right to left) Patrice Ficanos, Ploudaniel mayor Joël Marchadour, François Marchadour, and the late George Talec. Ploudaniel, France (June 2008). Photo by Susan McWilliams.

way through the hedges to the château, where two of our new friends from the toasting, the interviews, and the pork roast—Georges Talec and Daniel Berthou—walked us through room after room and related stories of the German occupation and how things changed in Trébodennic with the arrival of the 102nd evacuation hospital.

Now, back to August of 1944. The 102nd erected its tents adjacent to Trébodennic on the very pastures where the occupying German soldiers had set up their tents six days earlier. Dan, Ed Peterson, and Ross King bunked with Ren. With the hospital just a few blocks from the heart of Ploudaniel and its spiraling Église Saint-Yves, Ren and Dan "loafed" with the locals for the first few days and encouraged them to visit the new military tents in town. The 102nd physicians were not altogether happy with such visitors, but army directives called for this effort to build communication between "locals" and "visitors." "The chaplain [Kennedy] encouraged young children with their smiling faces and wild flowers to visit wounded soldiers" who were ambulatory, recalled Anne Vincot Bellec, "and doctors were not happy about it." If rules prohibited local visitors from entering the wards, Anne, "probably because [she] was an eighteen-year-old girl," received a rapid guided tour, during which she saw for the first time penicillin applied to open wounds ("We had never heard of it") and black GIs in the recovery ward ("We had heard of black people but never seen any before").

Likewise, civilians made use of the hospital. A young Resistance fighter accidentally hurt by a leftover German grenade received treatment for superficial wounds on one arm. Anne Vincot got "an injection" for acute asthma. Daniel Berthou, age nine, rode his bicycle into a tree as his eagle eyes followed every move of what the "new soldiers" called "football," which was being played at a small soccer stadium near the rear of the château property. Two hours later, "at the sound of a military truck," his mother, Jeannie Berthou, emerged from her spacious stone home adjacent to the château to find Daniel returning not on bicycle but in a 102nd ambulance, his right leg in a cast. "She did not know what was happening," recalled Daniel, "for the Germans had warned us they would return. Finally she saw the Allied insignia on the side of the ambulance."

These relative pleasantries, however, hardly filled more than a few days for Ren and others as the war and morale issues resurged. With ward tents still going up, indeed, in the late afternoon of Saturday, August 19, physicians McDaniel, Jennings, and Kunkel asked Ren to accompany them in a call on the CO to talk about the lack of "meaningful discipline" and people "not working together" in the outfit. He went. In the immediate sense the disappearance of the nurses prompted the visit: Was their wandering off the route on the way from Guingamp to Ploudaniel not just another sign of "disrespect and resentment" toward authority . . . the chief nurse? "Could the hospital function with nurses who could disappear?" The three understood at least part of Ren's assessment as given to Goodiel several days earlier. "What is wrong with the 102nd is the Chief Nurse and the Chief of Surgery." The CO promised change. Not expecting action, Ren went from the meeting to the tent of the executive officer, where, over "slugs of cognac" and accompanied by nurse Daves, he sought to bring Sutherland, as second in command, into the "conversation" about things not working. Two weeks later there was still no change. "[Physician] Ross King [after being] up all night operating [but still on duty] sat in our tent all day with [a] canteen of grapefruit juice and [medical] alcohol. Says he is waiting for Col. [Goodiel] to come in and tell him off . . . going to make an issue . . . demand an inspection." Sure enough, Goodiel had Sutherland investigate King, but "none of [the] witnesses [including

Ren] will testify that he was drunk." No investigation of Goodiel took place. And so it continued. "The hospital job is done well but [there is] constant beefing and bitching . . . [We] are wracked by dissension . . . [and] led by morons."

Despite no changes in management and morale, Captain King and his colleagues still had expanding developments from the war. Third Army HQ told Goodiel that the movement across Brittany and the liberation of Brest would be to "clean up" after prolonged and intensive Allied air attacks on the area. However, it turned out that the "clean up" involved thousands of casualties. There would be no time for films in the recreation tent. Ren chronicled the events. With sounds of "artillery getting heavier near Brest" and German planes sporadically strafing areas around Ploudaniel, by Tuesday, August 22, they were receiving about thirty new patients a day. August 26: "150 admissions . . . shock and pre-op tents full." August 27: "100 waiting for surgery." August 28: "200 new patients . . . put up additional shock tent." August 29: "All hospitals out here full—100th, 103rd, 107th, 108th, 53rd field hospital." August 30: "Running out of blankets, cots, tents . . . rain blocks air evacuations." September 1: "Man comes in with side of face blown off . . . dies on table . . . routine day." September 3: "165 [new] patients today . . . 30 or more hit by our own bombers." September 18: "Brest falls today . . . receiving German wounded prisoners . . . 250 of them by 10:00 PM. September 22: "Received 470 Germans at midnight." In the end, the month-long battle for Brest sent 3,000 admissions just to the 102nd, mainly GIs, but also a few French civilians and more than a few POWs. Fifteen died. Since the Normandy landing the deaths within the 102nd now totaled seventy-eight. Ren admitted: "I am tired . . . we all are tired."

Yet he still managed to pursue various nonchaplain inquiries—history, certainly, and increasingly medicine. When a break occurred in his rounds in the receiving and recovery tents, he followed his now standard practice of observing in surgery or pathology. "In A.M. I watched the most complete autopsy I ever saw. Dickey and Kunkel take out brains, lungs, spleen, stomach, intestines, heart, kidney" as they tried to determine what precisely had killed a GI. On another occasion, a GI "walked into ward [and] died 2 hrs later, no wound of any kind [showing]. Postmortem showed abdomen full of blood, holes in intestine, hemorrhage in all organs. The blast entered anus and blew him to pieces inside." Such postmortem insights wound up in detailed reports, as well as physicians' discussions and were immediately applied in keeping similarly wounded patients alive, a process the scholarly chaplain found "excellent." He also seemed captivated by surgeries risked to save lives. "I watch Capt Barrou bore two holes in a skull then he picks scattered bone out of skull." Nonetheless, the man died. "I watch Captain Dickey remove shrapnel from a kidney . . . interesting." The man lived. Two days later: "I watch Capt. Dickey operate on a scrotum, one-quarter of [one] testicle and one-half of the other are left." The soldier lived. Indeed, Ren engaged so many physicians in conversations about why they did what they did that, in the middle of the Brest battle, Sutherland—to get Ren out of surgery and pathology?—assigned him to develop assessments of GIs perceived as wanting removal from combat. The chaplain as medical psychologist. He thrived even picking up the medical jargon:

> A soldier with seven children shoots himself in foot; a good many SIWs [self-inflicted gunshot wounds]. I spend a good while . . . among combat exhaustions . . . These boys say they have headache, heart trouble, etc. According to theory most of them have none of these troubles but think they have [the troubles] to avoid going back to the front—not conscious of deceptions. [However,] some do have the trouble they claim.

A private came in with pain in his right knee—"injured nine years ago . . . he limps . . . Dodge says nothing wrong with knee [now] . . . it is a mental or psychogenic knee or hysterical knee (hysteria conversion) . . . set off by exhaustion." Of the 165 patients admitted on September 3, he concluded, "about half are CEs (combat exhaustion) and half are surgery," which helps explain the relatively low percentage of deaths among the patients admitted. Not surprisingly, during the month of September 1944 84 percent of CE cases in the 102nd were returned to action while 58 percent of "medical cases" went back to the front.

Just as intense if for other reasons was Ren's continuing exploration beyond the hospital. On September 11, with a significant break in the Battle of Brest—yet Brest was still some seven days away from full liberation—Ren and Dan managed to repossess *Alabama* from two physicians, acquire an expert driver from the motor pool, Private M. J. Anderson, and with no one's approval they drove straight down the D25 through the paused war and into *centre-ville* Brest. This effort "to see what damage was being done to the city" ultimately found them in a German-occupied sector under fire from rifles and small mortar. Ren undoubtedly froze in pure fascination with their predicament; after all, several folks back home had told him the war would afford him "good material" for preaching and writing. Dan, however, had the wits to suggest, "We should get out of here." With their only escape down a street clogged with blown-up tanks and trucks and no space to turn around, Private Anderson "backed the Jeep for a quarter mile," weaving through war debris—all accomplished "rapidly." Back at the 102nd that night the comrades toasted their escape with slugs of cognac. While Ren wrote his father that he and Dan had stupidly risked their lives going "to a place where we had no business," he smugly confided to the diary: "We were the first non-combat Jeep to get in" to Brest. Indeed, Ren remained so interested in what a totally blown-up city looked like—and that is what Brest was—that he returned with Dan on September 21, three days after the German surrender, and again on September 22 to tour the "foul" underground German hospitals from which some of the 102nd's POW patients had come: They came from "under a hell of rock."

On Sunday, September 24, Ren preached his twenty-minute morning service at Ploudaniel with a standard forty present in the Red Cross tent and then made rounds among the "probably twenty" patients awaiting evacuation. That afternoon, while "the men" took preliminary steps for the anticipated next move, Ren "loafed" with the locals and traded a carton of Lucky Strikes for two pairs of wooden shoes—the traditional footwear of Breton farmers. In the evening, having dropped off the shoe package at the Red Cross tent for mailing to Mary Conway and Margaret, he followed the Wilcox tradition of visiting with neighbors on a late Sunday afternoon. Since his first day in town he had been eyeing "the old French château squarely from [his] tent door," through which colonels Goodiel and Sutherland had made several courtesy calls. Now he walked up that hill himself and sounded the iron knocker on Trébodennic's massive wooden door. To the *noblesse,* Louis Croc, he explained that the 102nd was about to leave and that he was just dropping in to say "thank you" and to apologize for not having come by earlier to extend his greetings. Monsieur Croc invited him into the *grand salon,* where they sat down with his wife, Christine, his sister Marguerite, and his twenty-year-old nephew, Pierre Louboutin.

"Fresh pears and a bottle of Calvados" facilitated a "pleasant" two-hour visit in front of a seven-foot stone fireplace framed by shelves of books extending fifteen feet to the ceiling. That night Christine Croc noted in her diary—a dusty diary that Sylvie pulled out of an old desk and showed me—that the time with the chaplain was "very interesting." Ren heard the history of the great house from its 1584 origins with Alain de Poulpry, powerful counselor to the Parliament of Bretagne, to its partial destruction during the French Revolution and its reconstruction in the 1840s, to its purchase by the Croc family in 1850. He also learned of the striking contemporary life of the place. With their soldiers in tents down in the pasture, German officers had occupied the château for two years. These were not SS officers but the more civil Wehrmacht. Except for severely pocking all the floors with the nails in the soles of their boots and requisitioning Croc beef with deflated French francs, they did little damage to the Croc estate and left the family unharmed on their separate floor.

Still, fear, courage, and high drama ranged in and around the château. At 3 AM on June 3 the Gestapo arrested the celebrated World War I veteran and esteemed Ploudaniel school principal, Aimé Talec, for his Resistance leadership in the area; they beat him unconscious in the living room in front of his family, then dragged him away and tortured him ("asking for information"). When he divulged nothing, they deported him to the Bergen-Belsen prison camp in Germany. Yet, in the days after Talec's arrest—probably because of it—Louis Croc began providing "safe" space for periodic meetings of other Resistance workers in a room of the very house where the Wehrmacht officers lived—in Trébodennic. "Would the German officers ever think to suspect them *at Trébodennic?*" recalled Talec's son Georges. Indeed, at age nineteen, Georges had also worked with the Resistance, and when Louis Croc heard, shortly after Aimé's arrest, that Georges was next, he hid the young man in a "secret bedroom" in Trébodennic before passing him on to other safe places until the US forces could liberate Ploudaniel. "Trébodennic is a big place," Georges recalled. "The Germans never saw me."

From earlier "loafing" conversations—especially one with "a French woman [who had] spent 25 years in the U.S."—Ren had already heard a brief version of Aimé Talec's recent arrest and torture, as well as "other German atrocities" in Ploudaniel. He had also learned that Georges Talec, Pierre Louboutin, and other Resistance fighters had vainly tried to rescue Aimé during his torture time at nearby Rennes. But what the Croc family told him now topped all of this. Louis Croc concluded that evening with a discourse on the relative alcohol strengths of calvados, alambic (the

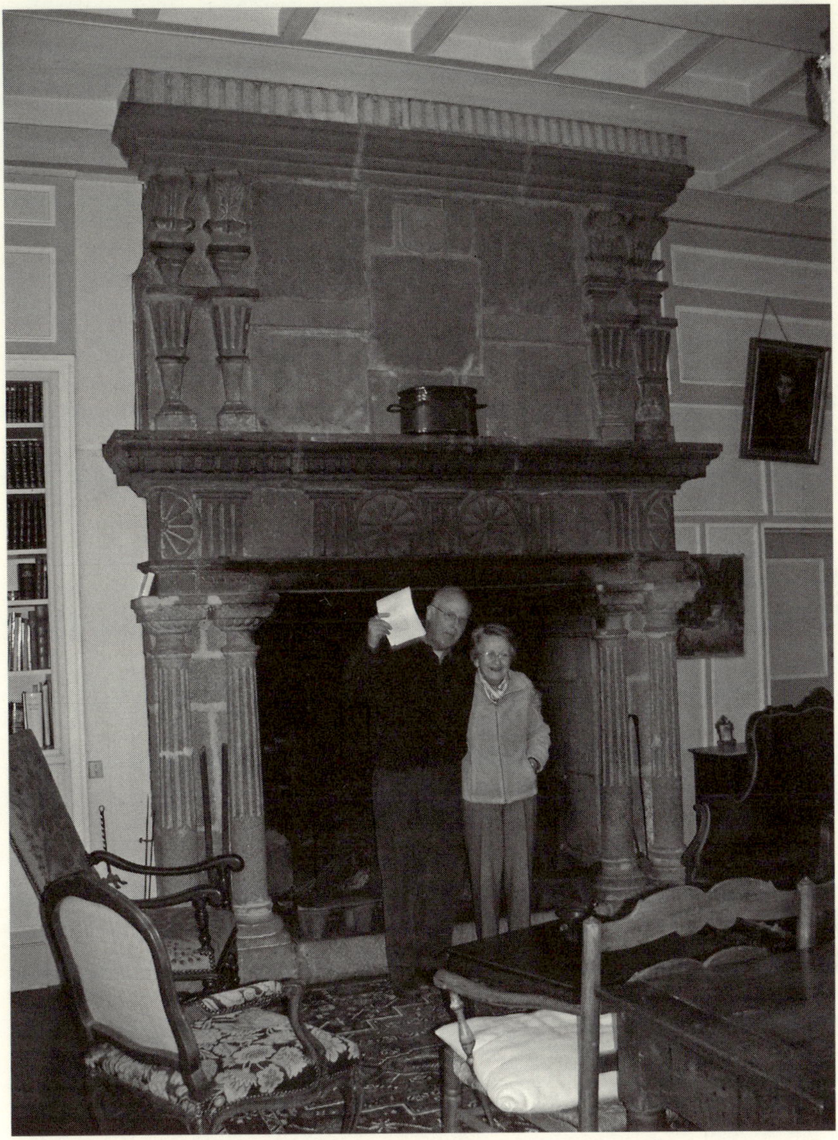

The author (left) with Sylvie Louboutin-Croc in the *grand salon* of the Château de Trébodennic, where, in September 1944, Louis Croc told RCK about Aimé Talec and other Resistance fighters and the German atrocities, Ploudaniel, France (April 2008). Photo by Susan McWilliams.

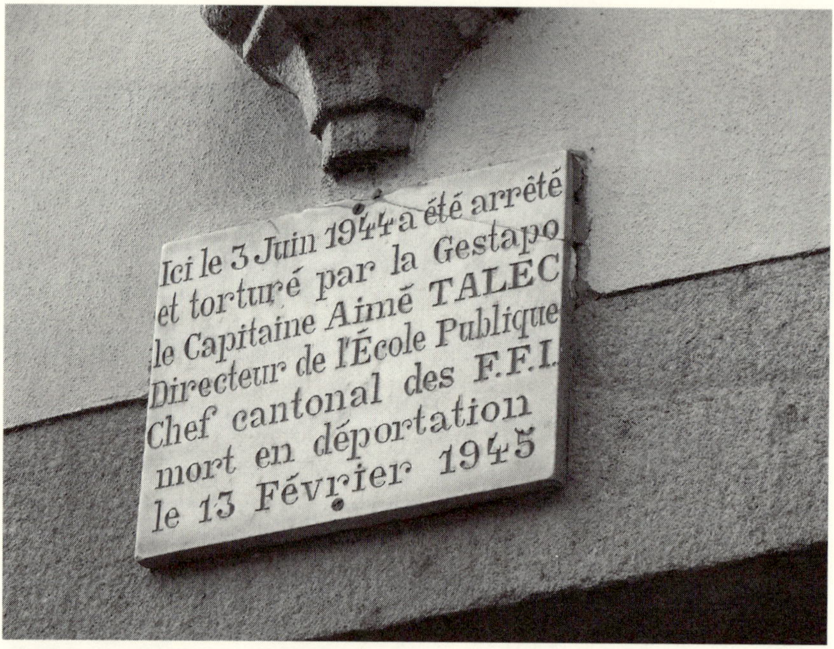
Ici le 3 Juin 1944 a été arrêté
et torturé par la Gestapo
le Capitaine Aimé TALEC
Directeur de l'École Publique
Chef cantonal des F.F.I.
mort en déportation
le 13 Février 1945

The historic marker honoring Resistance leader Aimé Talec, Ploudaniel, France (January 2008). Photo by Susan McWilliams.

Breton version of calvados), cognac, and *eau de vie*—useful information for a member of the 102nd. Then he invited Ren to come back.

So, the following night after an obligatory appearance at an officers' "cognac party," the chaplain returned to Château de Trébodennic with Dan and Ed as personal witnesses. Louis Croc gave them a tour of the place, pausing "at the historic points," then brought out his own (from Croc apples) alambic. Ren, Dan, and Ed had grown up in an American South rife with family Civil War stories about enemy soldiers in big houses. Some of these stories were true, others not. The Southern tales, however, seemed "diminutive" beside the five hundred years of true Trébodennic.

For the next two days, while the CO awaited directions, Ren worked with Roland to break down and pack the chaplain's office and the portable pulpit. With *Alabama* and the covered trailer ready to go, he settled into what he had not done since arriving at Utah Beach. He continued his new interest in sea stories with William McFee's classic *Casuals of the Sea.* He also experimented. After reminding Dan that Monsieur Croc had warned them about "the very potent" nature of *eau de vie* (60 percent alcohol), the two indulged in taste tests of the clear brandy, as well as Cointreau, cognac, and the far less potent cider. Nothing extreme.

Along with colonels Goodiel and Sutherland and two other physicians they had a more sophisticated time hosting Monsieur and Madame Croc at a 5 PM farewell turkey dinner under the tent. Their first time as guests at a seated dinner in their own pasture, the Crocs found it reasonable that hospital sheets could double as white tablecloths. The after-dinner entertainment, however, of the 102nd's vehicles driven around fast in a circle as if they were "cowboys riding around on motorized horses in a rodeo" they did not fully comprehend. Nor did their dinner partner, Ren. Still, Commanding Officer Goodiel "beamed with pride" at the spectacle, and gentle aristocrat Christine Croc proclaimed it "amusant mais très bon"—amusing but very good. When the vehicles finally came to a halt and the audience stopped coughing from all the dust in the air, Goodiel concluded the evening with an announcement that the 102nd was now headed toward Germany—to no one's surprise. This was followed by a toast to the Croc family for its hospitality.

At 7 AM the next morning, Friday, September 29, the 102nd pulled out, leaving "many" crates of "tin-can food," "boxes of condoms" (Anne Vincot Bellec: "We had never seen *préservatifs*—we were Catholic"), two broken trucks, and one Jeep. That afternoon, Christine Croc observed, the Resistance leaders allowed the locals a "controlled pillage" of everything left in the pasture, including items that lacked the pope's endorsement. Meanwhile, *Alabama* rolled along three back from the lead in a thirty-vehicle convoy of Jeeps, trucks, and ambulances. Roland and Ren took turns driving with Colonel Sutherland in the rear. Reassigned from the Third Army to the Ninth—and the entire Ninth Army made this trip—they headed east. They headed toward Paris, liberated on August 25, toward Brussels and Antwerp, liberated on September 4, and toward Luxembourg, liberated on September 11. But in this same direction also lay far more war, the battle for northwest France and Germany, which had commenced on September 12. They went to Bastogne.

The seven-hundred-mile trek—at forty miles per hour—took four days, with nightly bivouacs in still more pastures. They drove back through Morlaix, Guingamp, and Dinan, then on to Alençon and Mortagne, where they caught a view of Versailles. Bypassing Paris, the convoy went on up to San Quentin and Mâcon and finally crossed into Belgium at Givet on October 3. Temperatures ran unseasonably cold, and the rain rarely stopped. Much like others, whether in tent or Jeep, Ren dressed in layers of recently issued winter clothing: cotton US long johns covered with woolen British long johns, then a woolen uniform followed by a field jacket, trench coat, and a woolen blanket (a woolen overcoat came later). So attired, he motored up through France on his forty-fourth birthday. He wrote Mary a report about the big day, Sunday, October 1, 1944: "Get up in the rain and my bed was wet and I was wet . . . but sun is shining now and my bedding is dry. Travel in Jeep cold . . . taking the wind in a Jeep . . . Enjoyed the day in spite of rain and cold. A group of us ate one can of your birthday cookies last night." No mention of birthday or cookies, however, made it to the diary that night. Today he "saw many poor French, dirty ragged children, very frail and pathetic. . . . [They] hold up 2 or 3 eggs for sale . . . 10 yr old boy in answer to my question says, 'Papa prisoner in Germany five years.' Hold service in open at 3:30 PM. . . . 10 minute scripture and prayer." With each day the adventure became more complex and in fact more than complex as the cold and wet fall gave way to the brutal winter of 1944–1945.

PART THREE

Belgium, Luxembourg, and Germany

In the spring of 2008 Adam Pinson came to visit us. At the time an advanced graduate student in history at the University of Alabama at Birmingham, Adam has a long-term photographic memory. While this permitted him to trounce key contestants from Duke and Princeton on the television show *College Jeopardy,* from which he walked away with $50,000, it also facilitated his *minutely detailed* knowledge of World War II battles. With my needing him on battles and his needing Europe, we struck a deal: He covered his airfare out of "the *Jeopardy* fund," and we covered most of his other trip costs. We picked him up at the de Gaulle airport in Paris and gave him a day in Pennedepie to recover from the flight before spending two days at the D-day sites, where he saw, touched, and smelled what he had long had in his mind. Then we headed for northern Europe. Susan and I had been working historical turf of profound human dimensions. Now, with Adam knowing precisely where Patton's Third Army was on any given day and sitting on the back seat telling us about it (Pennie the Yorkie beside him, nodding approval), we followed the 102nd into some of the most dramatic military dimensions of the war and into places where the unit experienced its most trying times.

CHAPTER 8

Bastogne and Roumont

October 1944–November 1944

Bastogne caught us off guard. Ren left precise accounts of the 102nd's move there in the month before the fateful battle, plus numerous details on the town after the fighting was over. He actually went back to see it after Patton's "rescue" of the 101st Airborne. While we found plenty of places to buy miniature tanks, 101st Airborne T-shirts, and color photos of Patton, however, except for several small museums and the appropriately profound monument on the hill, the actual interpretive historic preservation at Bastogne paled beside what Ren wrote and what one might expect for the place where the two greatest armies in recorded history had engaged in one of their climactic clashes. You may say, "But the place was destroyed by history." So was colonial Williamsburg.

In the opposite way we also were surprised when we arrived at the heretofore unheard of—*except* in Belgium—Château de Roumont, where no battle took place but the 102nd functioned for six weeks. We expected to find no town, not even a village; if lucky, we might discover the remnants of a once-grand country estate. Instead, we eventually made out in the dense fog the outline of something rivaling Cornelius Vanderbilt's Biltmore estate in Asheville, North Carolina. With the proven cold knock on the door and the hearty "Bonjour!" we also found at Roumont the grandson of the distinguished entrepreneur and diplomat who had owned the château at the time Ren was there. Too, we found his engaging wife, Régine, their children, plus a superb roasted chicken and extensive family archives—even file folders labeled "US Army—102 Evacuation Hospital."

The serendipitous nature of human relationships, I suppose, made Château de Roumont even more unforgettable. Within a few minutes of meeting Jean-Christophe Coppée I told him I was from Birmingham. That afternoon as we parted, he said he knew something about Birmingham. In expanding Coppée Coal, Inc., of Brussels, his father had contracted with Rust Engineering of Birmingham in the early 1960s to develop their engineering unit. "Mais, oui, monsieur." Soon I was on the telephone with Alice McSpadden Williams of Birmingham, with whom I had grown up. I asked whether my memory was right: Did she and her husband, Tom—a Rust engineer—not live in Brussels in the 1960s? "Indeed, so," replied Alice. "Baron Coppée [Jean-Christophe's father] loved my fried chicken so much I excused myself from the table and went back to the kitchen and fried another one. He said he did not mind the wait. Those people in Belgium are kind people, quite social without being stuffy—in that sense like Southerners." (Two years later this serendipity continued. At a local political gathering back in Birmingham I ran into my seventh-grade teacher, Frances Poor, whom I had not seen since 1956. On hearing of our recent adventures in Belgium, she queried out of the blue: "By any chance did you meet the Coppée family? When my husband and I were in Brussels in the 1960s on the Rust assignment, the Coppées and everyone else in Belgium were so kind, so welcoming.") Precisely what Adam and Susan and I found, and precisely what Ren had found even if the 102nd as a unit did not exactly reciprocate.

On entering Belgium the 102nd was one of some twenty hospital facilities charged with taking casualties as the First, Third, and Ninth armies pushed toward Germany. The 102nd moved ninety miles northwest along the Meuse River to establish a holding operation in an upscale school facility in Bastogne. Created as a training facility for the German Youth Movement, then used by regular German soldiers until just three days before the 102nd arrived, the sixteen-building school had brick dormitories poshly equipped with real beds, multicolored tiled floors in the bathrooms, hot showers, oil-burning stoves, laundry rooms, and kitchens, indeed a "nicer army camp than any [Ren] was ever in in the U.S." While the 102nd awaited orders for five days—orders to be connected to reports from the new First Army action at Aachen, seventy-six miles to the east—Ren and his roommates, surgeon Robert Wassum and radiologist Sam Miller, relaxed with hot showers, clean clothes, and moderately consumed cognac. Ren and Roland took *Alabama* touring the "storybook . . . grand views" of the countryside, then visited central Bastogne to find a new band for the Lathan watch—"55 Bel francs or 67.5 Fr. Francs=$1.25."

While the chaplain recovered from the long haul from Ploudaniel, two negatives worked his mind: the outfit's continued lack of discipline and its poor management led to cases of stolen vodka flowing (along with nurses) through the officers' barracks. "Officers and nurses visiting promiscuously—a good deal of drunkenness." Since leaving the States he had seen heterosexual relationships in the 102nd come and go and even married one couple back in Southport. He had also been aware of discrete homosexual relationships among "the men" and "the nurses"—perhaps six in all—a few of which were whistle-blown (not by him) and sent home on CDDs. However, the overt lack of discipline he saw with the vodka drunks and the sex in the Bastogne schoolhouse bothered him for what it portended about the management of the unit and how this would play out when it returned to action. There is no indication that he tried again with either Goodiel or Sutherland.

"Sam Miller and I [just] stay in our room [and] Dan joins us." And this connected to his other "down" thought. As he wrote Mary (and he did not write her about vodka and sex), "I have never been as hopeful as some about an early end to the war. Seeing how these Germans fight and how well equipped they are has not been too encouraging. . . . The weather is already getting bad over here. I imagine there will be a big drive next month. . . . I will be in on the drive that is coming here." Prescience on both counts.

To free up the extraordinary Bastogne facility for the next strike against the Germans and to place the 102nd in "winter quarters" suitable for expanding casualties at Aachen, on October 7, 1944, the Ninth Army HQ moved the 102nd thirty miles west to Château de Roumont, just outside the village of Ochamps. The German officers had recently moved out. Ren exuded to Mary that this was "a magnificent building, 4 stories . . . I am [sleeping] on the 3rd floor with seven [other] officers . . . [and have] an office in an alcove under some stairs on the same floor." In fact, all of the male officers lived on the third floor, while the nurses were housed on the fourth, with some six bedrooms per floor. "The [enlisted] men," however, "did not get a very good deal": "stables [with] concrete floors which are cold and even after being scrubbed still smell like stables . . . A good many men have been to see me about it [but] it may be better in winter than we think." Despite the stairs, which made it difficult to move patients ("no elevator"), after relocating all of the first- and second-floor furniture to the attic, they converted the first two floors into hospital wards. The taxidermy stayed, however, and permitted the patients to gaze up at around fifty deer heads, twenty boar heads, plus pheasants and foxes. Another component of the second floor stayed, too—the chapel in the tower—much to Ren's initial excitement.

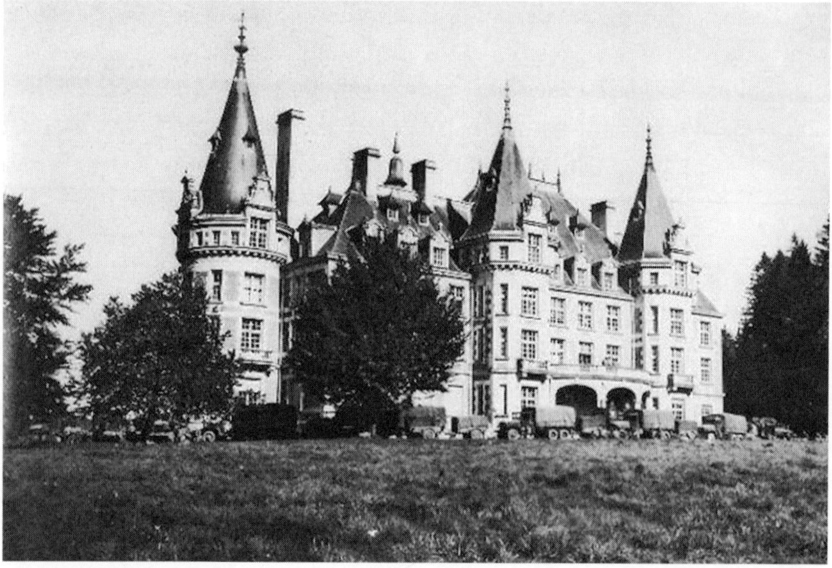

The 102nd arrives at Château de Roumont. Ochamps, Belgium (October 1944). Photo by RCK in RCK Papers.

For six weeks the 102nd stayed at Château de Roumont. Most of this time proved deceptive in terms of what lay ahead. Because evacs closer to Aachen wound up handling most of the casualties from that fighting, through the first week of November the 102nd rarely had more than fifty patients at a time, and there were no intense Ploudaniel nights with fifty wounded men stacked up in the shock ward. The temperature gradually moved down, and it rained a good bit. Significant snow waited until November 9, however, and the massive coke furnace in the château kept things reasonably warm.

With the patient load so low, Ren returned to some of his pre-France chaplain's life. On Sunday, October 8, at 10:00 AM he held services in the cozy chapel on the second floor. Virtually all of the forty seats were full to hear his "Why We Are Here" sermon. Moreover, that afternoon a Catholic chaplain, Col. Christian Wachter, came by at Ren's invitation so that the 102nd could finally have a Mass—a nice change after Ren's orchestrating ambulance transportation to local French churches for any Catholic soldiers who wanted to attend services. However, his ecumenical pleasure ended as the colonel, on completing his 4:30 PM service, "raised a protest about us using the chapel for Protestant services." Not knowing that the mother of Roumont's absent owner for much of her life had been a devout Prussian Protestant, Ren conceded to Mary that Wachter "probably . . . is technically right, but I told him it was a little narrow and intolerant and [a] contemptible attitude to take." From then on Ren's services were held down the hall in the Red Cross room—full thirty-minute services with regular sermons, piano music from Roumont's grand Steinway, singing, and good crowds—but "not in a real chapel."

"Local politics" also bothered him. A partisan Democrat, Ren set up his own presidential election bulletin board and counseled people on how to cast their absentee ballots. Still, the radio news of FDR's election in November gave "little local joy." As the 102nd's physicians razed Ren for being a "liberal" supporting "a socialist," Ren agonized over his doctor friends' "fearing they would not make a fortune when they got home" and being "a generation behind the social thinking of the country." At least one of them was also a thief. Ren had just mailed Mary a photo of himself standing next to *Alabama* when one of the doctors—"not sure which one"—stole the Jeep, leaving it wrecked in the neighboring village of Ochamps. "No one would admit who did it." With Dan's influence in the motor pool, however, *Alabama II* soon purred for explorations (still with "Alabama" painted on the front).

There was the Palace of the Duchess in Luxembourg ("delightful"), Verdun ("WWI memorials"), and Reims ("interesting champagne factory")—where Ren filled booze orders for the doctors. He also wanted to get down "near Nancy, France, " one hundred miles southeast, where Sam's armored unit was. Tough fighting there nixed the plan. Emboldened by Trébodennic, however, he indeed managed some personal social life at Château de Ronfay, two miles east of Roumont, where there lived, according to Roumont's resident manager, William DeGryse, a baron in charge of Roumont. Soon Ren was sitting with Baron and Baroness Hervé de Wykerslooth, mesmerized by their narration of the myth of Saint Hubert and their description of the hunting celebrations in nearby Saint Hubert. The baron must have found the chaplain engaging (or at least persistent). The following night, October 17, after a day in "stunning" Saint Hubert, Ren was back "next door" for supper with "the Baron and Baroness and their son Jack." At the table the baron complicated matters by explaining that he was not the real owner of Château de Roumont. That would be his wife's uncle, "Baron [Evence] von Coppée in Brussels"—the one with the Prussian mother, Ludmilla, and one of the foremost industrialists of Europe. The 102nd had landed in one of the most prestigious digs of Europe.

Few patients also created a fertile time for alcohol. Similar to life in most World War II evacs, in addition to cognac and other alcohol obtained locally, in the 102nd considerable liquor came one way or another compliments of the army. "Liquor allocation today for officers . . . one quart Vat 76 scotch, one-half bottle of gin" . . . at Roumont each week. Other alcohol, however, the physicians and nurses stole from the hospital with little or no objection by the commanding officers, notwithstanding specific army regulations against such activity. Ren had had encounters with "medical alcohol" beginning with the train ride from Bristol to Southport. However, at Roumont it flowed throughout the third and fourth floors from its "source" on the first floor as "grain," "ethyl," or "laboratory" alcohol, which was essential for any medical environment but especially necessary in pathology and postmortems. An average vodka was 80 proof; grain ranged from 100 to 200 proof. Upstairs they normally mixed it with pineapple or grapefruit juice or Coca Cola and with cognac for "serious" occasions. Regardless of the "formula," according to Ren's detailed cocktail notes, they called the drink "bug juice." Curiously, even unmixed or "straight," as in a dry martini—indeed, as in the infamous "Hawkeye martini" of *M*A*S*H*—it remained "bug juice."

Extensive bug-juice sessions occurred day and night. According to Dan's supply report, in one two-week period, while they averaged only sixty-five patients a day and had a total of three surgeries and no deaths or autopsies, the officers of the 102nd "used" thirteen gallons of medical alcohol. Surgeon Ross King and chief of surgery William Stewart competed for bartending accolades. Although Ren's regular roommates became steadfast friends on arriving in France, bug-juice bonding at Roumont escalated these friendships into the raucous life of a college fraternity—not available to Ren back at Erskine College. Dan's pronouncement that "this cognac [laced with grain alcohol] is *not* poison" swiftly became a quotable quote. In early November the seven even anointed each other with drinking names: physician Ed Peterson, "the Brain"; detachment commander Dan Laws, "the Brow"; physician Ross King, "the Pawn"; physician Tom King, "the Face"; dentist Robert Martin, "the Bull"; and chaplain Ren Kennedy, "the Pulse." Even beyond cocktailing, when two or more of the roommates were together, they "quit using . . . real names." Ren did not explain the origins of the nicknames. His would appear to be a function of so many members of the 102nd from the CO to "the men" coming to him for advice on life inside the outfit.

Despite his enjoyment in being "one of the guys" in bug-juice sessions, Ren understood the significant drawbacks to incessant drinking. Some folks regularly drank too much because of "personal problems" back home that they felt "powerless" to influence—"divorce" or the "death of a family member." The "powerless" problem also led some physicians or nurses professionally attuned to feeling powerful to "overdrink" after a particularly bad night with unending patients from the front. "Idle time" at Roumont, however, quickly had more folks drinking "far too much." "Since few read or have intellectual interests," the doctors and nurses had to be busy with the patients, and in Ren's mind the 102nd needed "200 to 400 patients" instead of the 50 at Roumont for everyone to be occupied. In that context, during October and November of 1944 the 102nd's management issues grew even worse. Constant drinking further eroded self-discipline, leading "some officers and nurses" to expand their "open sexual fraternization," which had begun at Bastogne. Realistic about outcomes, not to mention relevance, on Monday, October 16, Ren nevertheless gave his mandatory—once every three months—"sexual morality" talk to the eighty-five "men" who responded to the CO's "requirement." No doctors or nurses showed up. The "men" then asked Ren for a meeting at their barracks in the stables to discuss the unfairness of "rules and regulations being enforced" on them but not on others. The doctors and nurses, aided by a "stripe-happy" sergeant, continued to make them "do [personal] lackey service." While the "men" were expected to stay clear of sexual contact with the nurses, the physicians were not. Although the "men" were expected to be moderate in drinking their beer, cognac, and whiskey (grain alcohol was theoretically for physicians and nurses only), the bug-juice drinkers freely imbibed to excess. Ren explained the essence of the meeting to Goodiel. No optimism: "The Colonel has a tendency to promise many things and never do them."

Meanwhile, more "factions [and] cliques" developed as folks huddled after work for bug juice and griping. Nurses bitterly complained about Captain Ewing's "playing favorites with a few" nurses while being tougher on others. Physicians were equally bitter about Goodiel's delegation of key personnel decisions to a few "chosen" officers. He made 1st Lt. John Blackwell detachment commander in place of Laws, a defender of the "men." Then he let Blackwell, a nonphysician, trump executive officer Sutherland in determinations of which physicians would be sent for rotations at the front to give the field-hospital doctors recovery time at the 102nd. To Blackwell's credit, he managed to convince the CO to transfer the chief nurse, who, on November 10, moved to the 15th General Hospital

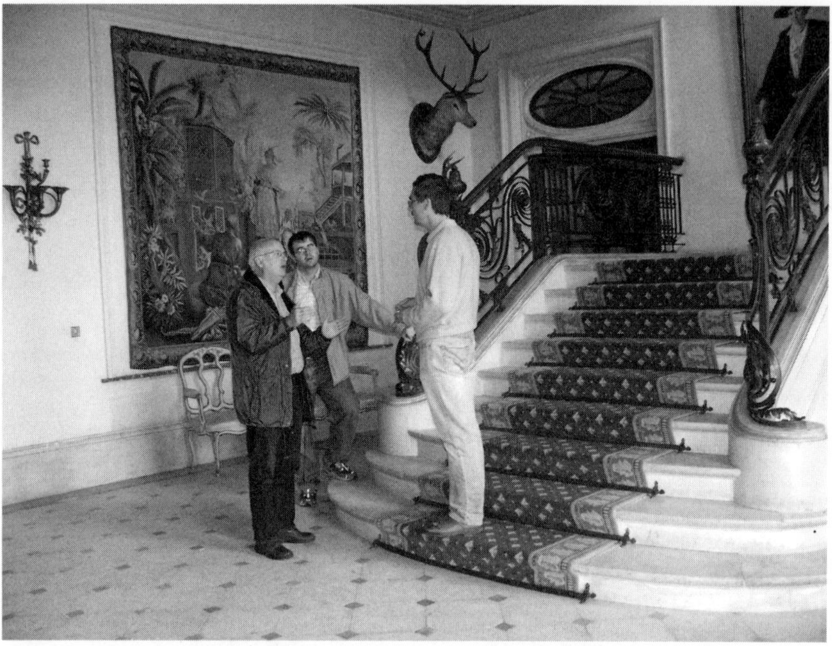

Jean-Christophe Coppée (right), Adam Pinson (center), and the author at the start of the grand stairwell inside Château de Roumont, discussing still-noticeable chips in the marble caused by rolling the physicians' beer kegs. Ochamps, Belgium (May 2008). Photo by Susan McWilliams.

in Liège. Ren hoped that a good leader would eventually replace this "old regular . . . Army" officer of "moronic incompetence." More pressing, within an hour after the chief nurse's departure, Ren somehow got access to Ewing's office and rescued his Remington portable typewriter, which she had confiscated four days earlier after another spat about her not letting the nurses go to chapel.

In the second week of November some of the key nurses and physicians held firm on wanting transfers, while others who wanted to stay but had crossed Goodiel and Blackwell found that they would be leaving. Regardless of the continuing bonds he felt with his roommates, Ren saw his movable "home" falling apart. Rumors persisted that Dan would be "eased out" to manage an ambulance company (which never happened). On November 15 "orders came through transferring [at their request] Nurse First Lt. Harriet Ayers to 2nd Evacuation Hospital and Maj. T. McDaniel to 67th Evac." On November 17 Major ___ Fincher received orders to transfer; he did not want to go and "cried" in a departure conversation with Ren. Others moved to temporary assignments in field hospitals. "I regret to see them go . . . breaking up of . . . congenial . . . Old Guard." That he exaggerated "the break up"—one or two physicians had moved in or out of the unit since billeting in Southport—as well as the unit's congeniality, reflected his deep engagement in the daily life of the 102nd. His analysis also captured the challenges of maintaining discipline, morale, and general momentum as the 102nd's greatest assignment unfolded.

After November 11 the 102nd played an increasingly important role when other evacs could not handle all of the casualties incurred as a result of Patton's push toward Metz. Still, as the 102nd found itself reassigned from the Ninth Army to the First Army, Goodiel received orders to move to a structure better suited for "semipermanent" wards and closer to the anticipated new front: the Ardennes forest. The 102nd was to move to the agricultural college in Ettelbruck, twenty miles north of the city of Luxembourg. On November 16 the personnel evacuated the remaining patients and started to pack. To Ren's deep concern discipline problems continued. "Men rolling [doctors'] beer barrels down stairs . . . break six fine stone steps . . . broken plumbing, lavatories, [electric] dynamo, furniture . . . cigarette burns in floors . . . It was a shame to turn this mob loose in it. . . . The Colonel and Blackwell never took any measures to protect it." First DeGryse and then Wykerslooth protested, emphasizing broken windows and irreparably pocked floors. Earlier, they stated, the exiting Wehrmacht Germans had tastefully stolen a few paintings and several mechanical parts for the furnace but were too disciplined to have wreaked such havoc on the great château. On November 19, after assigning adjutant Joe Rutenberg to stay behind to assess damages (about $25,000) and facilitate army compensation, Goodiel and most of the unit pulled out. The following day Ren and the few remaining officers headed to Neufchâteau and Arlon, then on to Ettelbruck.

CHAPTER 9

Ettelbruck

November–December 1944

Susan and I were accustomed to working in small villages and the countryside. Quickly we found that Ettelbruck was different—a small city in Luxembourg with complicated traffic. Our goal was the Ettelbruck Agricultural College; we had no specific address because, underestimating the scale of the city, we anticipated a huge complex that was easy to spot. Finally we got hand signals that meant, "You may be able to get there if you go down Avenue Lucien Salentiny." So, disoriented, we drove up and down this avenue several times until Adam shouted, "That's it right there on the right!" "How do you know?" "It's institutional looking—it was new in the 1930s, according to Kennedy, and look at those dents left all over the building from the small-arms fire." As the car moved to another angle, we saw the sign, large and obvious, guiding us to the main entrance.

Susan had been battling the traffic for us and said she would stay with Pennie. I was on my own with the French language—not bad in a market, adequate in a restaurant or bar, but inadequate for any complicated discussion. In we went. After "Bonjouring" my way to the director's office I was told that (a) yes, this was the right place and that (b) the executive assistant to the director, Monsieur Fey, could see us shortly. Ten minutes later a student assistant ushered Adam and me to a small office, where the bearded Monsieur Fey, age about thirty-five, sat at his computer dressed in jeans and an old sweater. "Monsieur Fey?" "Just call me Fred." Relief. Two hours later Adam and I left as the beneficiaries of a doctoral seminar presentation on Ettelbruck and the war given in Oxford-level English. You see, Fred was educated in computers and management, but his passion—what he would do if he could afford to go to graduate school—was studying the war. He was such a persistent researcher and careful writer that the Ettelbruck facility—now redeveloped as a technical college—had him writing a history of the school. Working online, he had delved deeply into materials located in the US National Archives. He knew all about the 102nd's stay at the college. Right there in Ettelbruck he downloaded and printed multiple documents from US military reports I had never seen. What he did not have was an hour-by-hour breakdown of the German assault on the school with the 102nd inside. We swapped details. And here is the whole story.

In May 1940 the Germans occupied Ettelbruck and converted the city's modern agricultural college into a center for retraining permanently wounded soldiers for agricultural work essential to the Nazi mission. When, on September 10, 1944, they fled the advancing US troops, the Germans left the four-story facility in excellent shape—minus the exterior walls, which had been dented by US small-arms fire, whose traces Adam spotted. Thus, forty days after its liberation the college became the 102nd's best situation yet for ward space (73,000 square feet) and was just six miles from the envisioned push into the Ardennes, which meant shorter ambulance time for patients to get back to an evac. At first there was little action. Ren inherited the college priest's fully furnished "fine" office with an adaptable living area ("privacy nice"). The nurses began functioning as a disciplined and cohesive team "almost exuberant" about their new leader, Captain Edith Bryan ("a very nice person"), who had arrived just before the move to Ettelbruck. Ren held brief Thanksgiving services in the officer's mess at 12 noon and another at 1:00 PM in the men's mess, then sat with Sutherland for turkey dinner. Although the facility had a chapel, he held Sunday services in the Red Cross room so that visiting Catholic chaplains had no complaints. Ren toured around. He found Luxembourg "about the size of Wilcox and Dallas counties back home," Bastogne still "beautiful." A physician known for having a bad drinking problem found himself transferred out of the 102nd for "medical reasons—patient [with] bad back." Five noncoms with similar drinking difficulties the CO transferred to a field hospital at the northwestern front, near Metz. Frustrated with Goodiel and his new detachment commander, executive officer Sutherland spent increasing time with his friends from SLO—"the Brow," "the Brain," and "the Pulse," who collectively baptized him "Pappy." The army provided an infusion of White Label scotch. Bug juice flowed.

Then life changed. First Ren found out about brother-in-law Sam. At supper on Monday, December 11, Flora Jane Bromley told Ren she had a Red Cross message for him. After supper he went to his office for open counseling hours, but he mainly just awaited the message. He knew what

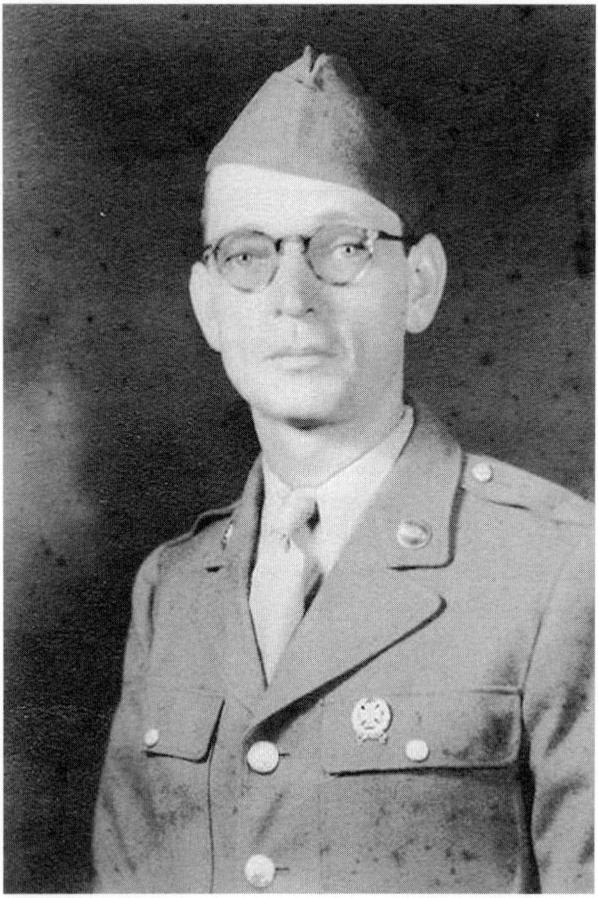

Pfc. Sam McNeill in April 1944, shortly before heading overseas. US Army photo in Sam McNeill Papers. Courtesy of Fleetwood Hollinger, Camden, Alabama.

Red Cross messages did. He just did not know who this one concerned. Finally, at 10:00 PM "she brings . . . [the] radiogram." It was from his sister-in-law, Dot McNeill, via "Washington to Continental HQ of Red Cross saying that Sam McNeill was killed in action in France on November 15. Saddest news I have ever received. It leaves me sick at heart." He closed his office door and walked upstairs and "just talked about Sam" with "Pappy." Granted, Ren had never been as close to Sam as he was with a few others back home. Sam was more of a "man's man," a devout hunter, fisherman, and deputy sheriff. He did not share Ren's obsession with the life of the mind. But the in-laws still held deep affection for each other.

From England to France Ren and Sam had stayed in vague contact with messages sent through Camden correspondence even though, with censoring, they rarely knew for certain where each was. Although it physically separated them, the war actually brought them closer as some of Sam's "man's man" tone gave way to something deeper. Sam had recently written Dot—a letter forwarded to Ren—that "how many Germans you've gotten will be more of a secret [after the war] than something to brag about . . . the man who really does these things is not going to talk so much." Then the strangeness of war brought them together in July at that intersection of country roads in Lower Normandy, permitting them several hours of "good catch-up talk"—war talk, the sharing of what news each had from home, and the all-important matter of boots. Sam had been trying to get Dot to order for him stateside a pair of twelve-inch-high waterproof leather boots from the L.L.Bean Company. Dot struck out. Still, with the strategic advantage of *Alabama* Ren said he could probably find them, given a month or so to hunt. Most recently, Ren sent word via Dot that he had located the boots in a shop in Saint Hubert, Europe's citadel of hunting, and mailed them to Sam. Even though the two likely were not that far apart, Ren had no idea how long delivery would take. But it did not matter now. The Germans had killed Sam.

The following day, after recovering some of his ministerial composure, Ren cabled his condolences to his sister-in-law; then that night he wrote her a long letter. Yet these were only "words," he vented to the diary. His own grief alone compelled him to do something else. So the compulsive researcher started a two-month quest to find out about Sam's death, starting with his own Red Cross message "to the Armored Division Chaplain inquiring about circumstances [of Sam's death] . . . and place of burial." This quest was complicated by an intensifying war.

Before daylight on the morning of Saturday, December 16, 1944, the Germans launched a carefully planned and surprising counteroffensive to the First Army's push through the Ardennes, starting what the Americans almost overnight called the Battle of the Bulge. Panzer divisions moved on Liège, Bastogne, Saint Vith, and Luxembourg city—where Ren had toured three days earlier. The initial attack barely slowed as the Allied air response struggled in intense snow and fog. Since arriving at Ettelbruck, the 102nd had had mostly painful trench foot (or "fat foot") cases from the 28th Infantry—dangerous infections on feet swollen by prolonged time in tightly laced, wet boots. Now, some six miles back from the initial Bulge fighting, the 102nd had the full engagement of a field hospital, plus an evac, as the Germans' heavy artillery hit all around the college from 5:30 PM on.

On Sunday morning, December 17, at 1:00 AM Ren finally left the wards. He managed to record the following: "Germans made an attack all along the front. . . . Hospital flooded with battle casualties . . . bad ones . . . over 200 admissions [with twelve deaths]." Well before daylight he was back in the shock wards, and at 10:00 AM he held a communion service in the Red Cross room: "37 present. Would have been a 100 but hospital overrun with patients." As Sunday, December 17, unfolded, the situation worsened. "Most deaths [in the hospital] we have ever had . . . many chest wounds. Patients all over halls [with] Germans [segregated] on second floor." When German soldiers took Diekirch, three miles north of Ettelbruck, the First Army command radioed Goodiel to relocate fast to its HQ in Spa, Belgium, eighty miles north. Just before midnight Ren tried to digest the pending crisis:

> [We] have orders to move 8:00 AM tomorrow. I spend most of PM packing. Rhynus and I load the [chaplain] stuff on the trailer. . . . Shells landing around here. . . . All patients evacuated this PM except 35 non-transportable cases [still being operated on]. Laws, Meads, Mills and [fifteen] enlisted men will remain with them. Shell fire and flashes and German planes tonight.

CHAPTER 10

Huy and the Bulge

December 1944–January 1945

What happened to the 102nd after Ettelbruck meant that Susan, Adam, and I next headed for Huy, a small Belgian town on the Meuse River, far easier for a visitor to navigate than Ettelbruck. Local tourist offices can be superb starting points—maps, kind people, and, for an English speaker, almost always an easy conversation. For fear of being spotted as tourists, many historians stupidly steer clear of them. We started there and quickly walked down the river to the facility once known as the Huy Normal School. We found a vast complex currently being overhauled for a multipurpose public space. The public library component was almost ready to open. That day we talked with construction workers. Later I found a local banker who was a first-class amateur historian of Huy during the war.

But you could envision it all at the time of the facility's *first* conversion—for the Battle of the Bulge: large rooms for wards; wide stairwells for moving stretchers up and down; a courtyard in the rear large enough to accommodate perhaps six ambulances; and nearby a former convent for yet more space. There is no monument in front of this complex. There should be—because here unfolded one of the greatest medical achievements of World War II.

The way the 102nd got to Huy was a lucky mess. When barely under way, Goodiel got word that the Germans were taking Spa. Either his subsequent orders were unclear or he did not follow them, for there "was much confusion, no one [knowing] exactly where to go." The convoy "got split up and wandered around for two days on Belgium roads." "Woojie" Schmittdiel's truck, loaded with "15 men," drove right by German tanks without incident, but three others were strafed by German planes. When another set of trucks found itself surrounded by German soldiers, a composed Sergeant Anderson—the same who had helped Dan and Ren escape Brest—urged the captors to examine what they were carrying:

hospital equipment only. The Germans let them go—minus twelve cans of fuel. In *Alabama* Ren and Roland stayed with the main portion of the convoy, which moved through Bastogne—three days before the Germans surrounded it—then went on to Houffalize and Aywaille, where they apparently got directions via the CO of the 67th Evacuation Hospital to head to Huy, sixty miles to the west, arriving there the night of Monday, December 18.

They piled into various rooms of the abandoned Huy Normal School and went to sleep. The next day, as its separated trucks slowly rolled in, the 102nd set up to function in the school as part of a rapidly developed hospital *center* in the school's four large buildings and in other Huy buildings, too, including hotels, a convent, and even a brothel vacated the day before. Ren walked around town. He found hospital units brought in from some one hundred miles across the front: the 68th Medical Group, the 44th, 51st, and 67th evacuation hospitals, the 3rd Auxiliary Surgical Group, and the 4th Convalescent Hospital, with twelve hundred patients.

Goodiel's unpopular detachment commander, John Blackwell, assigned himself to be Ren's new roommate. At 8 AM there was no heat inside, and it was twenty-one snowy degrees outside. However, indoors and with cots they were still significantly better off than lying on the ground in the middle of the Ardennes forest. Thursday morning, December 21, "after much anxiety and contemplation as to their fate," Dan and his two ambulances finally showed up, having had no choice but to flee amid intense shelling that was quickly followed by the Germans' retaking of the Ettelbruck facility during the night of December 20. With no choice in sight, the thirty-five "nontransportable" patients became "transportable." Miraculously, all made it. The same day the ambulances started bringing in casualties from the Bulge—299 the first hour.

Over the next five days the battle raged several miles away. Allied forces took a horrific beating. Granted, on December 23 improved weather finally permitted an effective Allied air response, which eventually turned the tide, but the catastrophic casualties kept up. The 102nd became "an insane madhouse" made even crazier by the "buzz bombs" and the "ack, ack, ack" of German antiaircraft weapons. Physicians, nurses, and "the men" worked combat shifts of twelve hours on, the same off. Bug juice slowed to a trickle. December 24—Christmas eve: "513 admitted . . . a line of ambulances at the front door waiting to unload and another line at the back door [through the courtyard] waiting to take them to a general hospital." Most—Ren carefully noted—were from the 82nd Airborne and the 3rd

Armored Division. This only increased the next day. On Christmas itself, 667 were admitted, 575 evacuated, and 150 operated on due to the Christmas eve "back log." At 8:00 PM 70 were still waiting for surgery. Then it eased. Despite "badly wounded from the 101st Airborne" who had just been rescued by General Patton's 37th Tank Division from their besiegement at Bastogne (from the same German Youth Movement facility the 102nd had occupied forty-two days earlier), on December 27 admissions dropped to 378, evacuations to 331, surgeries to 25. By December 31 admissions were down to 55, evacuations to 10, and surgeries to 10, "leaving no back log." That night Dan and Ren faintly signaled the New Year with a bottle of champagne. But there was no other celebration: "Bob Kunkel [a physician] receives word tonight that [his] 4 year-old daughter [had been] killed [back in the States], 3 other children and wife in hospital . . . automobile accident," which punctuated Ren's New Year's Eve "hope to be at home Dec. 31, 1945." In its last two weeks 1944 morphed into "a sad year." It was no longer "an adventure."

Indeed, on New Year's Day Ren was not encouraged by the fact that "the hospital [was] empty" and "the front in this area is quiet." The Germans could not have been beaten. He anticipated "a move." In the lull he was anything but buoyed. To his earlier inquiry about his brother-in-law's cause of death and burial site, he received a short response that gave "no information"; he forgot what the US Army actually had on its hands and railed to the diary about its "insensitivity" regarding Sam.

He showed the same uncustomary sense of reality as General Eisenhower's temporary reorganization of the First Army transferred out many of its senior officers, including the 102nd's CO Goodiel. Ren attributed Goodiel's move more to "his general ineffectiveness as a leader—[for example,] the damage done to the Château de Roumont . . . [and] the messy move from Ettelbruck to Huy"—and less to Eisenhower's recasting his leaders to avoid a repeat of the large-scale chaos in the First Army, which had given the Germans an advantage in the initial stages of the Battle of the Bulge. Ren probably was right, as Goodiel, on January 12, 1945, received a "Special Efficiency Report" that resulted in loss of rank and ultimately reassignment as a surgeon. (After the war Goodiel returned to senior army ranks with Legion of Merit recognition for his work in military disability and rehabilitative medicine.)

Still, in his admittedly "down" frame of mind, Ren looked upon the new command more as a sign that "the 102nd is steadily changing . . . no longer the old organization it once was." This inadvertently raised

Goodiel's stock—a little. Even if Goodiel "was kind of stupid and very inefficient," he nevertheless was "as good as [any of the] old regular Army officers . . . a good man and my friend." Likewise, when the new First Army command immediately named the CO of the 44th evac, Col. John F. Blatt, as temporary CO of the 102nd and, by January 2, 1945, had him managing the two units as one, Ren lamented: "I don't even know some of those who are coming in . . . 44th evac personnel . . . many strangers . . . roaming around the place . . . insolent, arrogant." In short, though his war "home" had actually been breaking up for some time, the intensity of the Battle of the Bulge and its "sad" consequences rebonded him to the 102nd, moving him first to re-create this "home" in his own mind and then believe "the Army" was taking it away. Captain Kunkel's leaving on January 3 to deal with his family tragedies in the States just made things worse, for they had been friends since Southport. "A good man." "May never see him again."

After four days the lull abruptly ended as the Luftwaffe sought to reestablish the German offensive in the Ardennes. Bombs and strafing produced a new wave of casualties inside the 102nd, which was still at the Huy Normal School. January 4: With some 223 admissions, 200 evacuations, and 22 backlogged in surgery, "we are now being used as a field hospital." German troops then broke back into Belgium and Luxembourg and decimated the American infantry. January 7: This battle is "about as tough as anything that has happened in the war . . . casualties enormous . . . too great to be published in the U.S." Although the German forces ultimately were unable to prevail in the Ardennes and began withdrawing into Germany on January 7, the casualties kept coming. January 10: "[O]ver 500 admissions yesterday, even more [600] today, the toughest since Christmas day." January 11: [M]any, many more . . . one a pilot . . . needed a bucket to bring him in." Finally, by Wednesday, January 17, admissions were "slacking" to 170, evacuations to 200, and the surgery backlog to 11. The Allies had won the Battle of the Bulge. Other components of that makeshift medical center at Huy bravely carried their loads and more. Still, the 102nd was the only one of them to have escaped the surprise German attacks of December 16–17 with its transportation and medical equipment essentially intact. As a result, of the 19,000 American casualties at the Bulge some 4,700—25 percent—received treatment during those eleven epic weeks at Huy at one evacuation hospital: the 102nd. Moreover, of those 4,700, only 100 died while patients at the 102nd.

Throughout most of the ordeal Ren maintained his standard chaplain duties. On Christmas Eve, Sunday, December 24, "so much turmoil" from the battle kept him from holding regular services although he managed "3 ward services for 200 men." However, on succeeding Sundays, January 7 and 14, he preached at 10:30 AM in one of the large classrooms of the school building ("How Germany Has Rejected God") with about sixty on hand. More important, like the others he worked twelve-hour days in the admitting and recovery wards, sharing individual communion services, Bible readings, prayers, and "just talk" with "those who regularly saw men blown to bits before their eyes."

Among these "brave and uncomplaining boys"—GIs as well as POWs—were Millard and Willard Lumpkin from Delta, Alabama (near Anniston). Identical twins, back in Delta they not only "shared headaches" but also corner jump shots on the high school basketball court—jump shots so identical that the coach could never tell which brother was on the court. As a sharecropper's sons, they had had to quit school after the tenth grade to take work at a pipe foundry in nearby Oxford, Alabama. On turning eighteen, however, they joined the army, eventually finding their way to Europe as part of the famed 83rd Infantry, 33Q Regiment, Company G. On Friday, January 5, 1945, at 7:30 AM—a good hour before daylight—the 83rd was attacking the German line at Rochefort, France, when Willard took severe shrapnel wounds to the stomach, chest, and limbs. Positioned less than ten yards away and with shrapnel wounds to his own right leg, Millard teamed with a medic to get Willard onto a stretcher and then carry him almost two miles to a field hospital, from which an ambulance took the twins and ten others to the 102nd at Huy.

While the surgeons worked on Willard that evening, Ren talked with Millard—the Alabama connection, the horror of the last day—while others dug the metal out of his right leg. Twice during the surgery Ren checked on Willard. Even though he shielded Millard from some details—"saw Vic Mills remove packing [applied by a medic] to Willard's chest and two quarts of blood run out"—he honestly reported the gravity of the "sucking chest wound." The surgeons ultimately emerged with little hope. When Ren took Millard in for a visit, they found Willard lingering on heavy doses of morphine. Well after midnight Ren told the diary the following:

> Willard died at 12:30 AM [January 6, 1945]. Sgt. [Leonard] Reichlin shaves him, combs his hair, puts him on the table with blanket over him, face exposed—looked nice. I take Millard in to see him and say prayer. The

> twins born August 17, 1923 . . . The mother Mrs. Ethel Lumpkin, Rt. 2, Delta, Alabama. [Willard will be] buried at Fosse, Belgium.

The next day, January 7, with Ren's help, Millard wrote his mother:

> Willard died Friday night. . . . It seems that I cannot do without him. I am left alone but someday I hope to meet him. . . . he lived 17 hours after he was hit in the right leg and right side. . . . Captain Kennedy from Camden, Alabama, was there with us at the hospital. It was hard to give him up but we had to do it. He was put away nice. I will get by some way.

Three weeks later back in Delta, Alabama, Ethel Lumpkin, with her young daughter Maudine, walked the mile down the dirt trail to their mail box facing Mount Moriah Church Road. Ethel was thrilled to find two letters from overseas. First she opened Willard's—a censored, upbeat account of war news mailed two days before he was hit. Then she opened Millard's. "She just fell down," recalled her daughter, pointing at the ground. "She almost died right there in *that* dirt."

"Sucking chest wound" was just one of many medical terms Ren continued to pick up as he "finish[ed] each day" with a now well-established battle pattern of "an hour or two in the operating room at night." Yet "evisceration of abdomen," "trench foot," and "paralyzed diaphragm" now were more than new vocabulary. With "medical adventure" gone from his mind, they were the core of traumatic life in war. January 11: "This insane business keeps on." January 12: "This horrible war." January 13: "Men suffering and dying around here all the time . . . it gets more and more sickening."

Amid such tragedy and trauma, this intellectual chaplain began describing his feelings as being in a "brown," a term depicting deep thought about death and the fragility of life he knew well from one of his favorite poems, John Crowe Ransom's "Bells for John Whiteside's Daughter." Yet this reach for aesthetic expression of his situational depression in no way diminished his anger and frustration. His longtime criticism of "the Army" hierarchy lost all balance. On January 8 Goodiel's permanent replacement arrived: Lt. Col. John R. Woodruff, a senior surgeon from the 9th Infantry. Although Woodruff was the first "new Army" CO to manage the 102nd, Ren ignored the upbeat possibilities and let Woodruff's appearance take him further "down," down below worrying about the 102nd as a dissipating home and on down to his most intense and sarcastic attack on "the Army" and its prospects for victory:

> Just another stupid regular Army blockhead, I don't know. I can't say much for the regular Army people. . . . There is not much quality to most of them. Maybe that is why it takes so long to win the war. They are the fellows who get all the promotions and make the plans and run the war. I can't escape the feeling that if the Germans had had the men and equipment we had they probably would have pushed us into the Atlantic Ocean long ago. Certainly they gave the Army a terrible beating for about three or four weeks. . . . I don't think we have made a good showing in this battle, but the fault has not been on the part of the dough boy, the individual soldier. He has done his part and done it well. . . . News of Russian drive in Poland is good . . . Maybe Russians can win the war for us.

Breaking news about Sam's death temporarily eased the "down." Sergeant Reichlin's mortuary duties included transporting those who died in the 102nd to the closest US Army Graves Registration Unit. On one of these trips he advised Capt. Thomas A. Roundtree of the 612 QM Graves Registration Company at Ménil-la-Tour, near Metz, that Ren was looking for Sam. On January 18 Roundtree relayed through Reichlin that Sam was buried at Limey Cemetery between Metz and Nancy in northwestern France. If the final fighting between Limey and Huy kept Ren from asking permission to take off a few days to visit this site, the immediate prospects for going held out at least something positive and concrete he could do amid the otherwise chaotic tragedy. His morale began to recover.

The next night, Friday, he wrote his first relatively "up" lines in the diary since December 18: He was pleased that "11 people" attended a rabbi's service he had arranged for the Jewish personnel, and "Bruce's juices" (bug juice) with Dan, followed by "steak supper," were "good." The depression continued to ease. In the late afternoon of January 20, while still "sick seeing the boys come in . . . suffering, dying," he and "the Brow [Dan] had a canteen of bug juice" while studying a map and the complicated route to isolated Limey. The next day, when "the new Colonel Woodruff" (now "a nice fellow") granted permission for the three-day round-trip run to Sam's grave, Ren even experienced a short-lived change of heart regarding George C. Patton. The one he had so vigorously vilified nine months earlier for his "utter vulgarity" suddenly, after huge victories in Belgium and Luxembourg, would possibly "win the war for us. [The 102nd] was in Patton's army [from August to October of 1944], and I liked it better than this one." So, if Ren still "wanted to come home, and stay" and the Ardennes battle remained "a bloody and terrible thing," he told Mary, by January 22 he had nevertheless recovered some of his enthusiasm for the army and the bonding it had always provided: "Today is Dan Laws's birthday—26 years old. He comes to my room in PM and we celebrate with bug juice. I give him ten cigars."

At 9 AM on January 23, with Dan unable to get off, Ren and Roland headed *Alabama* for Sam's grave. Eighteen inches of snow on the roads kept their speed under twenty-five miles per hour; despite heavy woolen clothing and blankets, the zero-degree temperature made them stop twice at POW camps to warm up. After feeling their way through Verdun and Saint-Mihiel they finally reached Commercy, France—twenty miles from Limey—and spent the night at the 50th General Hospital. The next morning, after the confounding discovery that Limey was not the precise location, they ultimately pulled up to the US military cemetery, situated one mile outside of tiny Noviant-aux-Prés. Just as Captain Roundtree had promised, there was Sam. Ren offered an extensive funeral service despite the brutal temperature and falling snow. They then drove twenty minutes to Ménil-la-Tour, where the 612 QM Grave Registration Platoon provided "data" on Sam's death—how and where he was killed. After another overnight at the 50th General Hospital the two headed home in subzero weather, detouring slightly to check up on Château de Roumont. Somebody's bombs had "shattered the tower" with the chapel, but otherwise the place was the same—chips in the marble steps still offensive. Back in Huy that night, January 25, Ren typed Dot a lengthy letter undoubtedly to help not just with her closure but his as well:

> I sent the [two] Graves Registration men back to their tent. Then Rhynus and I placed our helmets on Sam's grave. I read the 23rd Psalm and some verses from John 14 and [we] repeated the Lord's Prayer. Then I sent Rhynus back to the tent and I stayed out there by the grave with Sam for a half hour just thinking about him and talking to him. I had no flowers in this terrible winter over here. But I cut a small evergreen limb from a fir tree and placed it and a copy of the Gospel of John opened at the 14th chapter on the grave, and weighted them down with a lump of frozen clay. Then I said another prayer and left. From the cemetery we went 10

> kilometers . . . to the office of Graves Registration. . . . I learned [that] Sam was killed in action on November 15 [1944] at a place called Béchy, France [twelve miles southeast of Metz on the east side of the Moselle River,] from [mortar] shell fragments, wounds in head and chest. It is probable that Sam was killed instantly or at least was never conscious after being hit. . . . He did not go to a hospital. Had he lived for a few hours the medics would undoubtedly have picked him up and started him back to a hospital. They get the man out as quickly as possible even going under fire to pick them up. Many medics have been killed doing that. So I think it is likely that Sam was killed instantly and if he had to die I am glad it was that way for I have seen the terrible suffering of many of the wounded. [His] grave has a wooden cross, white, at its head. To the center [of the cross] is nailed one of the identification tags a soldier wears. The other is wrapped in waterproof material and buried with the body. . . . The Report of Burial Sheet was dated 17 Nov 1944.
>
> In the spring and summer it must be very beautiful in this section of France. It was beautiful yesterday, too, in a way, covered with twelve inches of snow. Sam is not sleeping there alone. There are 5800 other American boys sleeping there with him, and there will be some more. . . . I think of Sam every day that comes. . . . It must have been close to zero down there yesterday. But I would have gone if it was forty below for Sam's sake, and yours, and also my own.

To this letter he attached sketches laying out the cemetery, plus a map showing the way to Plot J, Row 9, Grave no. 209.

Over the following two weeks, as patients became fewer and fewer, Ren regained a degree of his pre-Bulge spirit. Granted, "the Army" returned a difficult package to him. The Saint Hubert boots he had mailed Sam came back to him in an "unfeeling return to sender" box. Though they were a full size too large, he just decided pragmatically that he would wear them himself—no army angst or heightened sentiment. He also joined more than a few of the rapidly reappearing bug-juice sessions, chortled over Dan's "liberating" a case of Coca Colas from the PX ("genuine Coca Colas and they are good"), and renewed his subscription to *New Republic.* He wrote Mary not to send any more grits, for "our food is good and plenty of it. . . . I probably weigh eight pounds more than I did when I left home." When Mickey Rooney made a USO call at Huy, Ren managed a personal conversation after the show. The comedian had "a bad sty" on his left eye, "had not had a haircut for two months," and looked "like a bum," Ren explained to Mary, because he "traveled in a Jeep [giving]

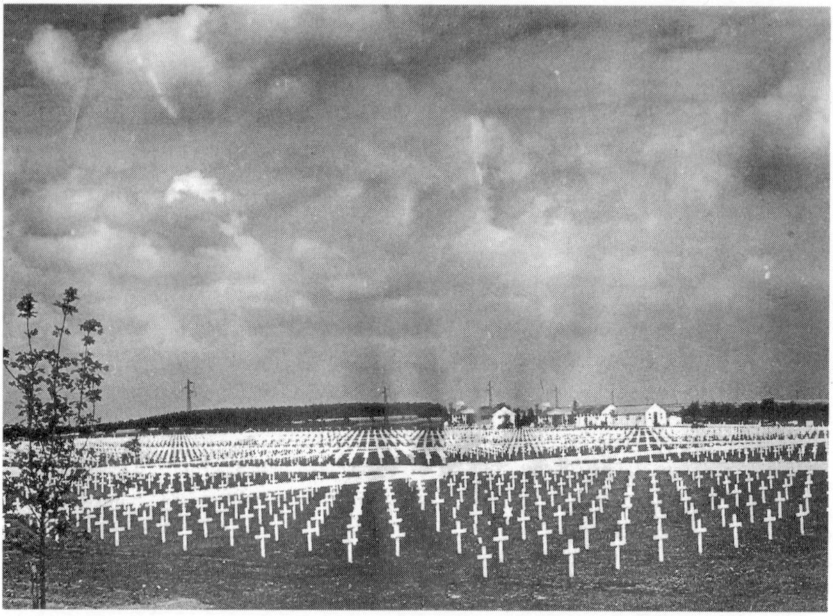

The temporary graveyard for US soldiers created just outside of tiny Noviant-aux-Prés, France, where, on January 24, 1945, RCK found the grave of his brother-in-law, Pfc. Sam McNeill, covered in snow. US Army photo (c. 1946) in Sam McNeill Papers. Courtesy of Fleetwood Hollinger, Camden, Alabama. As of 2008 this location was a massive agricultural site with no marker indicating what had happened there in World War II.

sometimes as many as four shows a day" to provide "good entertainment" for the troops. Woodruff's stock also continued to rise: "A very nice person . . . good enough to me."

But his negativism was far from gone. When the 102nd received confusing orders about when it would move out for its next assignment, Ren pounced: "This Army . . . stupid." Then, somehow overlooking Patton in the Ardennes, "I have never seen any job that civilians could not do easier, cheaper, quicker, and better than the Army does it." Most important, even though he granted that "the Army" was winning the war despite its flaws, his sermon on Sunday, January 28 (sardonically titled "Victory!"), reflected an overarching cynicism. As drafted on small sheets of USO stationery, his message began with the reminder that all "our hopes on entering the war" focused on a "world federation, the end of imperialism and [the] rebirth of freedom." But "what has war done for our [own] country? The slaughter and crippling of 1,000,000 [US] soldiers." And "what has war done for Europe? Freed [it] from Nazism and Hitler but not freed it from fear, want, savagery, tyrannies, and despair." He predicted that after the war Europe would exist "as two spheres of influence, Britain's and Russia's, not unified." Russia would have "Finland, Poland, Bulgaria, Rumania, Yugoslavia, Hungary, Czechoslovakia, Austria." Britain would have "France, Holland, Belgium, Portugal, Italy, Greece, maybe Spain." Ironically, as with World War I, "Germany will be the prize." If Britain's "sphere" failed to balance Russia's, "there could be [a] communistic government in every State in Europe in ten years except in Scandinavia, Switzerland, and the UK."

He concluded with little concrete optimism. Contrary to the hopes of many, "the war does not [after all] give us a better chance to rebuild the world; [it is] better that we had started that in 1920." To avoid total "despair," therefore, Christians should "face" this repeated debacle with "intelligence, courage, righteousness and repentance," and somehow their values could assist the postwar world in averting "chaos." In short, "the Army" was not alone in being flawed. All of World War II was flawed. In this less than uplifting Sunday morning message—undoubtedly one that his CO wished had not been delivered—the chaplain implicitly rejected his own longtime pro-war stance. Yet beneath the futile geopolitics, his feelings also were deeply personal, religious, and oppressively "brown." There were the Jews, the Finns, and the Poles. There were Vasco Hale, Bleuette Bindel, Aimé Talec, Willard Lumpkin, and certainly Sam McNeill, not to mention the hundreds of thousands of others poignantly admitted to the wards of the 102nd—Allies, Germans, civilians. The tragedies that befell these otherwise everyday people had ultimately gnawed down Ren's once strong engagement of war—patriotism, adventure, indeed religious duty—to one vague and muted marrow of Christian hope.

CHAPTER 11

Brand and Bad Neuenahr

February–March 1945

Susan and I had two days left with Adam, our traveling companion with the photographic memory. After that he intended to go solo and explore German beer parlors and war museums and then spend several days in Paris before flying out. We headed south, still with Ren—to sorrowful Dachau and then to Hitler's Eagle Nest. So, for those two days we focused on the 102nd's next major involvement: with the Allies' taking of Remagen Bridge, just inside Germany, and its treatment of casualties at the nearby Kurhaus Hotel. First, we visited what is left of the bridge and its small but excellent museum while being treated to a compulsively live narration by Adam Pinson. Then it was on to one of Germany's grandest hotels. Although the lobby of the Kurhaus is filled with photographs that tell its history back to its nineteenth-century origins as a spa, this visual record lacks any reference to World War II. The kind, professional staff said they had never heard that their establishment had been a hospital during the war—no doubt a story lost when the original family owners sold out to a Europe-wide corporation in the 1960s. But one thing is certain: At least one US soldier, Renwick C. Kennedy, never forgot that it was there, inside the nurturing Kurhaus, that he began to climb his way out of the "brown" of the Bulge.

On Thursday, February 1, 1945, after forty-six days at Huy, Commanding Officer Woodruff moved the 102nd out of the Huy Normal School into the convent two blocks away, which other US Army medical units had been using. The change permitted the 18th Corps to establish operation in the school complex while positioning the 102nd for its next move in support of the Allies' crossing the Roer River—the final western assaults on Germany. On February 4 the 102nd motored fifty-five miles just inside the German border to Brand, near Aachen, and set up in a former German cavalry school. For four weeks the hospital treated casualties from US troops pushing on across the Roer and Rhine rivers. Other

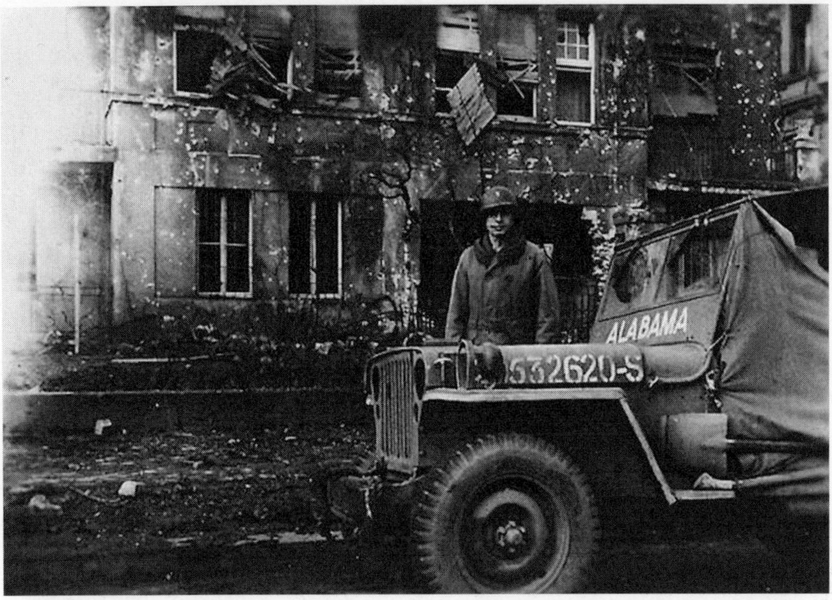

RCK and *Alabama II* in blown-up Bastogne, Belgium (March 1945). Photo by Roland Rhynus, courtesy of Rolinda Rhynus Luevano, Colton, California.

wounded soldiers included those who had been felled around Remagen on March 7 and 8 as German 88s futilely responded to the US troops' surprise taking of Ludendorff bridge across the Rhine. Despite "Jerry planes constantly overhead," a "lot of ack, ack, ack," and "12 dead in the hospital," on March 4 the casualty load in the 102nd was "at least half" that of the Battle of the Bulge. Hence, in some ways Ren's life returned to "normal." *Alabama* took him and Ed Peterson sightseeing in blown-up Liège and Bastogne. He methodically visited patients in the wards and offered Sunday services. He counseled one member of the 102nd on his pending divorce and two others who were being sent home for homosexuality. He observed surgeries and postmortems. Virtually every evening either bug juice or scotch lubricated small gatherings of lengthy, serious talk. In addition, CO Woodruff reorganized his staff so that two of Ren's good friends returned to "power"—Basil Winstead to executive officer, Dan Laws to detachment commander. Yet this "normalcy" set in the growing hours of "beautiful" sunlight and daytime highs in the midforties did not reverse the fatigue, stress, and sadness. On February 24, returned to his role as chief of surgery, Colonel Sutherland—increasingly Ren's "good friend"—sent word that the chaplain should stop using hymns in Sunday morning services, for they interrupted the "medical meetings in next room." His diplomatic skills worn to the nub, Ren ignored him. "We sing hymns anyway." February 28: "Everyone tired." March 3: "I am tired," and, despite recent promotions for Basil and Dan, "Old Guard whittled down." March 4: "sweating out Sam's letter" (hoping the censors had not blocked the long letter to Dot). March 9: "Lt. Strom invites me to go with him to Paris," where Ren had never been—"I decline"; and March 10: big bug juice gathering, but "I do not go." In place of large social settings he preferred the serenity of recently arrived back issues of the *New Republic* and *Christian Century,* as well as Dorothy B. Hughes's sad new mystery novel (converted to a Hollywood film in 1943), *The Fallen Sparrow,* which probed Nazi power and the death of innocents.

Patton's Third Army, Bradley's First Army, and Montgomery's Operation Plunder kept moving beyond the Rhine, and Soviet troops coming from the east targeted Berlin. So, on March 14 the 102nd loaded up the trucks and again headed east 134 miles to Bad Neuenahr, just north of Bonn. "The men" wound up in tents, but the officers and patients landed extraordinarily well. Just leased by the Allied command, the Kurhaus Hotel was a nineteenth-century Wilhelminian-style resort that normally offered guests "spa healing" in the warm mineral water that bubbled up from adjacent volcanic rocks—one of several noted spa bath (*bad*) facilities in the area. Yet, even in this otherwise uplifting environment, the war did not go away. The 102nd inherited a large patient load from the 45th Field Hospital, which had gotten to the Kurhaus a week earlier, and during the transition Ren happened upon "a German girl [who] dies in a ward . . . [with] vomit and blood in her mouth . . . because no one was there." Over the next twelve days every time the hospital evacuated its patients, it immediately returned to at least 50 percent capacity, surgeries on "25 bellies and 25 chests" a day not uncommon. Saturday, March 17, saw special drama when the collapse of the liberated Remagen bridge killed twenty-eight US soldiers, and the surviving forty casualties arrived at the Kurhaus; the next morning almost no one attended Ren's Sunday service because "everyone was too busy . . . very, very busy . . . with the casualties [from] the collapse."

Still, in this place Ren rebounded—up to a point. Though war closed the recuperative spa, he marveled at the "tremendous building" and luxuriated on the second floor in "a private room with chairs and a bed with a soft mattress" that doubled as his office. Undoubtedly comprehending how rest and decent surroundings can influence one's perspective, he confided to the diary his discovery that the German word for "cure" is *kur,* as

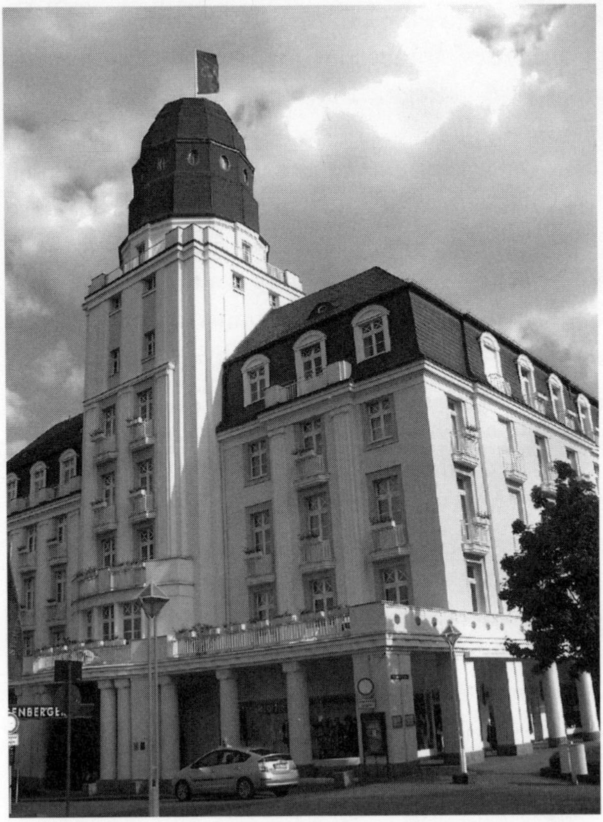

The Kurhaus Hotel, where, in March 1945, the 102nd treated patients from the battle for the bridge at Remagen. Bad Neuenahr, Germany (May 2008). Photo by Susan McWilliams.

in *Kurhaus.* Before long he was focusing on the "clear and beautiful days" and his perception that Bad Neuenahr was "a nice town" and mentioned that the "trees [were] just beginning to put out leaves."

Then Colonel Woodruff gave him his "efficiency report." Although Woodruff had quietly told him on several occasions how valuable his "counsel" was on various issues, the timing of such a formal written appraisal could not have been better. "A sincere, understanding officer with an outstanding sense of diplomacy," wrote the colonel, "[a person] capable of handling the most delicate situations . . . gaining him the respect and admiration of all persons contacted." Ren's spirits rose. He was elated to load captains Golden and Rutenberg into *Alabama* and make the short run to neighboring Ahrweiler "for the first service [at its synagogue] in ten years" since the Nazis had shut it down. He enjoyed conversations with "a fine Negro chaplain" who was in and out of the Kurhaus, checking on casualties from "a Negro infantry division." Indeed, as he moved back "up" his morale concerns seemed limited only to "probably too much bug juice" and "cigarettes" among the officers, including himself. On March 18, while the 102nd struggled to treat the Remagen bridge casualties, a group of "visiting brass . . . colonels . . . getting drunk with their women, their nurses" in several hotel rooms generated much griping and low morale among "the men and the officers," but it did not return him to the "brown."

By March 28 battle casualties admitted to the hospital had slowed to "a few a day," and freed US POWs—soldiers captured at the Bulge—began arriving. In an afternoon bug-juice session with Ren and a few others Colonel Woodruff stated flatly, "The war is over." That was premature. Still, three afternoons later Ren sipped "choice bug juice" as he optimistically reviewed his sermon for the upcoming Easter Sunday. First developed for an Easter back at Camden in April of 1941, the sermon ran some eighteen handwritten (7" × 9") pages. Nothing suggests that he tweaked the proven message for wartime (as he had done on other occasions). It was just a standard, eloquent Kennedy talk about the reality of resurrection—not vague hope—framed by Matthew 28:6 and Judges 13:23 and interlaced with humanistic quotes from Shakespeare. When he gave it on April 1 he felt particularly good: "Pretty Easter. A.M. chilly but sunny. I hold 3 ward services for 28 men and have an a.m. service [outside in a tent] with 110 present, one of the best services I have ever had in the Army." This was so different from Sunday, January 28, back in Huy.

The difference continued that afternoon. In *Alabama* he took Roland and S.Sgt. Loren Gill sightseeing. With a sense of adventure remindful of the dangerous Brest escapade they were "unable to get into Cologne [as] MPs stop us on three [different] roads." Even though the Allies officially took Cologne back on March 7, they encountered "artillery and small arms fire around Cologne—east bank still in German hands." Still, they moved on to Bonn ("beautiful") and visited the home of Ludwig von Beethoven before returning to the Kurhaus via new pontoon bridges across the Rhine at Remagen. Along the way "peach, pear, plum, pansies, violets, shrubs [were] in bloom." Compared to the recent past, Easter 1945 was indeed good.

CHAPTER 12

Final Days in Europe

April–October 1945

With complicated thoughts left to be finally sorted out, Ren's war resumed. The 102nd followed a rapidly moving First Army in the final days of fighting in Germany. On April 7 the hospital set up in tents some two hundred miles farther east at Warburg ("an appropriate name"). The diminishing war permitted officers the option of billeting in town. However, because of the damage to Warburg, most of them, including Ren, found the pyramidal tents (after a two-day search for five hundred lost tent pegs) more accommodating. For the two weeks in Warburg they averaged 70 in the wards per day from actual ongoing battle and military vehicular accidents and another 250 a day from Allied POWs recently liberated from German camps—soldiers from "Scotland, US, Russia, Belgium, New Zealand, Italy, Australia, Poland, France . . . emaciated soldiers," Ren emphasized, "in many cases nothing to eat at all for six days" before reaching the 102nd. Still, compared to Huy and even the Kurhaus, the schedule of the 102nd relaxed. And the now predictable consequence of downtime reappeared. When Ren's Jeep first rolled into Warburg, its covered trailer brought along gallons of medical alcohol and cognac. Only at Roumont did bug juice flow the way it did at Warburg as doctors with hangovers constantly struggled with nausea and diarrhea. As a result, "surgery is just moving too slow," Ren observed, "nothing like Brest [Ploudaniel,] when we were at our best."

On April 21 the 102nd moved another 150 miles east to Gera. There, as German forces in the Ruhr surrendered and the Soviets reached Berlin, the liberated POWs—especially Yugoslavs, Czechs, and Rumanians—continued to flow steadily into the hospital. In other ways, too, the Warburg pace continued. After a sleety and rainy first day, the oil heaters were used less and less in the tents, the days were "clear," "fine," and "beautiful," and outdoor bug-juice sessions pondered when it would be all over.

Ren had time to explore the town, where stockpiles of German military goods turned up in warehouses. Along with many officers from the 102nd he visited several of these sites. Although he expropriated a cavalry saddle envisioned as a gift for daughter Margaret, a subsequent memorandum from First Army HQ reminded him that such behavior was illegal, so he returned it. His self-avowed "moral laxity" in the chaos of an ending war was "appropriately corrected."

Other adventures gone bad were more difficult to correct. One drunk private accidentally shot another drunk private. Still another drunk private fell off a truck and was run over and killed in the traffic. In addition, three of "our truck drivers . . . drunk . . . run over 3 liberated Hungarians, killing one and breaking arms and head of another [then] pull .45 [pistol] on [our] warrant officer." Ren did the funerals. Out-of-town travels included two trips 220 miles northeast to the Buchenwald concentration camp, the first trip on April 25, just two weeks after the Allies liberated the horrific facility. After seeing "a few prisoners" still in the camp under treatment from US field hospitals, he returned to Gera with two fundamental thoughts: "So many Jews killed . . . SS so very brutal."

Although back to being adventuresome, he still was in this reflective mood when, on May 8, the radio brought news of the German surrender. He was naturally "up" about the war winding down. "V DAY IN EUROPE!" he began his diary entry. "I hear speech by Churchill at 3:00 PM [on radio]," and "I hold Victory Day service outdoors . . . singing [as per army directive] 'Faith of Our Fathers,' 'Star-Spangled Banner,' 'God Bless America,' and 'My Country, 'Tis of Thee.' Good service." But the celebration did little to dim the war's still unfolding reality: "4 deaths in hospital last few days, 2 [of them] DOAs, a Russian . . . [and] Lt. Roy Crooks of Concord, North Carolina, fractured skull, 3/4 ton truck wreck, died this AM." On further reflection about the day—after the Victory Day service—"everyone was quiet and cared little for noise."

Gradually heading toward their exit from Europe, the 102nd reversed course on May 13, when it moved two hundred miles toward the Rhine River. Again they set up in tents—this time in an alfalfa field outside Giessen, thirty miles north of Frankfurt, where they stayed for three and a half months although the hospital actually shut down after July 19. Rarely did the cots have more than a hundred patients, normally some eighty of whom were liberated POWs from every army imaginable. The remainder included a nurse from the 102nd, who broke her collarbone while stealing home plate in a softball game, and a flow of various US Army personnel who got drunk and accidentally shot each other or wrecked a Jeep or a truck on the autobahn.

Ren occasionally watched surgeries and postmortems. June 12: "I watch Dickey for 2 hours do post mortem on [Arkansas soldier who died after a motorcycle crash] . . . drunk, ride motorcycle standing up, waving to girls, shouting Heil Hitler." After daily ward visits he offered the usual counseling in his tiny tent-office. The only unique case was a "very tough one." Six "men" of the 102nd found themselves accused of raping two girls, ages fourteen and eighteen, back in late March at Bad Neuenahr. At the CO's request Ren spent hours with the accused, first in his office, then in the Giessen stockade, seeking truthful information and counseling them on the legal proceedings they were facing. In France such accusations against GIs could have led to jurisdiction by local civilian authorities and death by hanging. Courts martial, however, ultimately sent the majority home on dishonorable discharges for vague involvement in the matter but not before "a boy from Arkansas with a complex personality" confessed to explicit guilt in both rapes. He explained that people believed he was homosexual when he was not. In the stockade two days later, "somehow [he] stole a pistol" and "shot himself in the heart—dead." After holding a "subdued" funeral at 0900 in front of the tents, Ren joined the CO in leading a short, formal officers' meeting on the significance of the death (there is no record of their conclusion), then wrote one difficult "condolence letter" to the boy's wife. Otherwise, his work in Giessen offered little out of the ordinary.

Now that the workload was relatively low, Giessen provided opportunities for more exploration in the Jeep. There was the "dark, long, sad" trip to Dachau. Here Ren visited his brother, William, whose last combat assignment in World War II was lead physician with the 10th Field Hospital, where he provided medical treatment for the liberated. William recounted what he had seen. Ren stared at "lamp shades made with human skin." However, he also had uplifting and interesting trips: a "fascinating" visit to Hitler's Eagle's Nest, where mighty *Alabama II* scaled one hell of a mountain in first gear at seven miles per hour, and to his general staff hideout at Ziegenberg. None matched the "Jeep's eye view" of Paris with Dan in mid-July, however, which was facilitated by another liquor run for the doctors. With the Jeep pulling "a one ton trailer . . . we stop at Reims . . . champagne factory to see about liquor. PVT Carl Brooks [their driver] stops Jeep too close to railroad tracks and a passing train tears

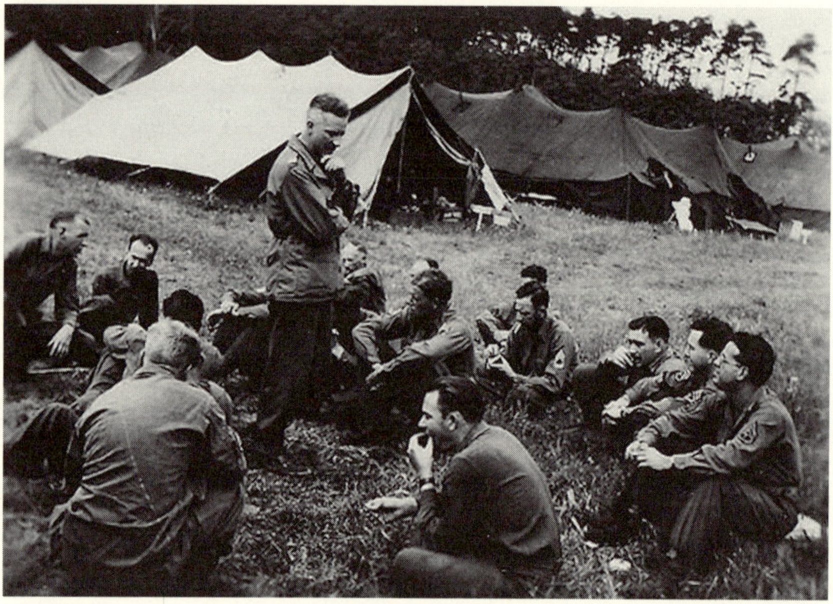

Col. John Woodruff, CO of the 102nd, addressing officers after the suicide of the soldier who confessed to raping two German girls to prove to his comrades that he was not homosexual, Giessen, Germany (June 1945). Photo by RCK in RCK Papers.

whole windshield off, hits Brooks['s] nose. Could have killed us. We get Jeep fixed at [neighboring US Army] Ordnance . . . leave trailer and go on to Paris." "Billeted at Rhone Hotel on Rue Jean Jacques Rousseau," they sampled Paris: "Arc de Triomphe, Champs Élysées, Eiffel Tower, Latin Quarter, Notre Dame, Versailles . . . the Louvre . . . Bastille Day streets full of people . . . American Church, beautiful building, sorry sermon . . . Chaplain (Maj.) Ira C. Frazier murders English language." Finally, after three days they got down to their assignment: liquor. "July 16—At Reims. Get [one-ton trailer filled with] champagne and liquor. Laws drives [back to Giessen] after accident in Reims."

Despite engaging trips and on June 30 receiving one of fifteen Bronze Stars awarded to the 102nd's 350 personnel, Ren shared his comrades' frustration as "the Army" worked by fits and starts to bring the American troops home. June 9—"No news about what will happen to us"; June 16—"102nd [is] classified Category 4 which means go home and be discharged"; June 30—"People restless . . . wondering what will happen"; July 18—"We landed in France one year ago today"; July 19—"Hospital closed. Just sitting here in this field . . . hot, uneventful." Unsurprisingly, along with kimmel, champagne, scotch, and kirsch, the bug juice gained even greater currency once the hospital shut down. Though hardly ones to deny complicity, on at least two occasions Ren and Dan carried "just smashed" doctors back to their own tents late at night. Yet, the waiting also permitted immersion in classic literature: Stephen Crane's *Red Badge of Courage,* Konrad Heiden's *Der Fuehrer,* William Shakespeare's *Macbeth.* These widely different perspectives on conflict, courage, and moral order provided an "intellectual marinade" for his reflections on life since joining the 102nd back at SLO.

This situation continued on July 30, when Colonel Woodruff received orders to move the 102nd twenty miles northeast to Marburg and reopen the hospital in a former German military barracks. There, Ren and others learned of Japan's surrender, but the chaplain's exhilaration dissipated when he was assigned to counsel yet another enlisted man facing legal procedures after a battered fifteen-year-old German girl accused him of rape. Otherwise, if now far removed from a "brown," Ren's "restless . . . bored . . . frustrated" mood persisted as "the Army" tried to work its way through the chaos of "going home." In August he found himself inexplicably joined by two other chaplains, Winter B. Luckett (Catholic) and Lawrence R. Davis (Methodist)—three chaplains for a three-hundred-person unit.

Chaos "advanced" when the Allied command moved the 102nd from the Third Army to the First Army and CO Woodruff was sent to another evac and was replaced by a recent Harvard medical school professor, Lt. Col. Grantley W. Taylor. The First Army then reorganized the 102nd's "officers and nurses" to report up through the neighboring 41st Evacuation Hospital while merging its "men" with the 70th Division—then after four weeks it countermanded this change and left the 102nd in tact. Unable to comprehend what was going on around him—in reality, the complicated drawdown of the largest military operation in history—Ren saw these changes as ineffective bureaucracy by "the Army!" and representing "no progress at all toward our going home." Indeed, even as his desire to return to Wilcox County intensified, this "full disorder" ignited a resurging need to hold on to the 102nd as "home." On the night of Thursday, August 30, he proudly recorded in the diary, "The Pulse, the Brow, the Bull, the Brain and the immortal Barfield and Buckley had a real party—never to be forgotten."

On September 10, when Woodruff departed, Ren lamented the loss of this "very good guy of the 102nd." Although he was not one of the 102nd's

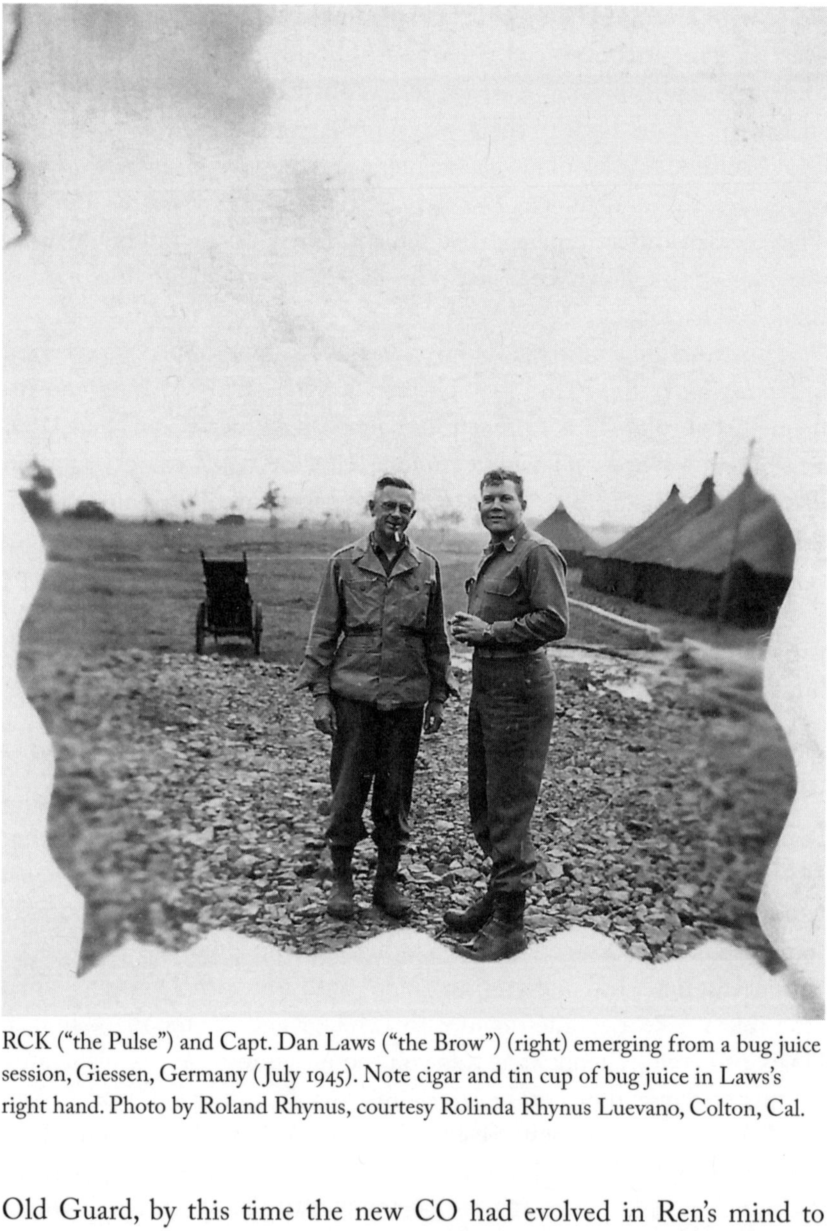

RCK ("the Pulse") and Capt. Dan Laws ("the Brow") (right) emerging from a bug juice session, Giessen, Germany (July 1945). Note cigar and tin cup of bug juice in Laws's right hand. Photo by Roland Rhynus, courtesy Rolinda Rhynus Luevano, Colton, Cal.

Old Guard, by this time the new CO had evolved in Ren's mind to "a good guy" who approved the chaplain's absences for sightseeing and lent his pet cocker spaniel, "Cokie," as "shotgun" for *Alabama*'s continual beer runs around Marburg. Ren vented that Woodruff's replacement "should have been" long-time medical chief "James Jackson Barfield." This "subject" kept the Old-Guard bug-juice sessions, usually hosted by Ren in his spacious private room in the barracks, running full force. They waited and waited. They slept so much during the day that Ren obtained "sodium amytal" from his physician friends to enable him to sleep after dark. On September 3, when substantive word finally arrived that they actually would head home in three weeks, Ren spent the next week writing a fourteen-page "History of the 102nd Evacuation Hospital." Later published as a model "unit history" from World War II focused on SLO, Southport, Ploudaniel, and the Battle of the Bulge, here was his typically clean-cut prose, except for concluding lyrical lines, where he turned maudlin: "A salute to the 102nd, a salute with a tear in our eyes from those who loved her best." He omitted many personal thoughts.

On September 19, "our last day in Marburg," Ren completed packing, spent "an hour" in town "just watching the people," then went to a tame party for the Old Guard in the room of nurses Betty Baker and Hazel Middleton, who had been with the 102nd, too, since SLO. Things were less tame the next couple of days. The 102nd rolled out of Germany and headed for Camp San Antonio in the sprawling Reims (France) Assembly Area Command, where they were to await redeployment. Dan rode in the Jeep with Ren. Roland drove. As they overnighted at the army barracks at Metz, Dan somehow took possession of Ren's diary—the only time during the war when another person wrote in it. Dan still had the day's liquid momentum in him: "Today we were on the B.J. [bug juice] at 10:00 A.M. At 7:00 PM we were still chewing out majors and other field grade officers. This has been one of the roughest days in the history of medical warfare. From here to New York harbor its [*sic*] anything short of a general court martial and more Juices of the Bug." Ren—not deleting anything—appended a more sedate note: "Travel in convoy today. Rains hard at times. Laws and I ramble around the camp [at Metz]."

The next day, September 20, the 102nd pulled into Camp San Antonio. In this tent city eighty-five miles west of Paris they merged with some two thousand other GIs who were sooner or later headed for home via Marseilles or Le Havre. Much like his 102nd colleagues, for the three weeks at Camp San Antonio Ren had no structured duties though he occasionally assisted with church services. Because his one-man tent had no electricity or heat, he spent the daylight hours on his cot covered in blankets and reading classics checked out of the tent library. Thomas Wolfe's *Look Homeward, Angel* gave him "pause about what it will be like after the war in Wilcox." Poker, bridge, the World Series via radio, and movies took up nights, as did bug-juice gatherings. When the medical alcohol left over from Marburg finally ran out (October 5: "Laws and I mix our last ounce of bug juice today . . . no more, first time in a year"), occasional army rations of scotch and gin kept the gatherings going but at a much lower tempo. In between books he and Dan took off on farewell jaunts in the Jeep. Now well acquainted with Reims, they made a "champagne procurement" run to the historic champagne factories—"avoided another train mishap"—and spent an hour at l'École professionnelle de Reims, the city's technical school. Here the 101st Airborne was resting when it was suddenly called to Bastogne. Here General Eisenhower had established the Supreme Headquarters for the Allied Expeditionary Forces. Here also, the German High Command had signed the German Capitulation Act, ending the war in Europe ("tables and chairs there with names of men who sat in them.") Indeed, Ren's increasingly revitalized sense of European adventure kept his morale "generally up" even while he was surrounded by buddies frustrated over "no news" about a precise exit date.

That date got a lot closer after October 12, when the 102nd convoyed sixty miles south to another of the Reims assembly points, Camp Baltimore, adjacent to rail lines headed on down to Marseilles. Although it was another tent city, it boasted electric lights throughout, even in the library, which stayed open until 10:00 PM. For seven days Ren "lived" at that library, where he sat engrossed in old friends from Shakespeare: *The Tempest, Julius Caesar,* and *Romeo and Juliet.* Then, on October 20, the 102nd, minus its trucks, Jeeps, and hospital gear, joined the 2nd and the 97th evacuation hospitals, plus "an engineering outfit" to comprise a ten-car freight train ("1000 people aboard") bound for Marseilles, five hundred miles to the south. After pondering how "*Alabama* [now] has left me," he went to "sleep all night cramped up on a seat . . . no glass in window . . . cold."

They wound up in yet another tent camp at Calas, ten miles outside of the port. The tents lacked electricity, but the camp library had lights, and the army ran regular buses into Marseilles, which was all Ren needed to make the most of "exiting Europe." He divided the next twelve days between library reading—Somerset Maugham's new *Razor's Edge,* depicting war trauma—and port-city adventures. He found Marseilles "old, dirty but right interesting: all kinds of people . . . loaf at sidewalk café, sip beer, eat raw oysters with bottle of vinegar and glass of wine . . . watch people—all kinds—U.S., French, Moroccan, soldiers, sailors . . . a cross-roads world city." Most folks around him in the tents "got down hearted" when on Saturday, October 27, word arrived that they would board ship in two days, then found that this "alert" applied only to the nurses at an adjacent camp. Ren, however, showed little frustration. He caught a bus to Marseilles "to see the nurses off." Finally, at 10:00 PM on November 1 the chaplain looked up from his diary to see his beaming buddy at the tent door. "We have been assigned to a ship, the *Porpoise*," Dan proclaimed, "and we leave in two days." This time the bulletin proved true. The next day, Friday, Ren packed his bedroll and footlocker, then attended a "last night in Calas" gathering for remnants of the 102nd evac, details unrecorded.

A C-3 transport carrying twenty-seven hundred troops, the USS *Sea Porpoise* ("What other kind is there?") eased out of Marseilles at 4:30 PM on November 3. For the next ten days the vessel chugged along at its maximum speed: eighteen knots. Intermittent rough seas left Dan and many others of the 102nd continually sick. Blessedly immune to seasickness, during the day Ren escaped the "suffocating" air of his room below, shared with sixteen other officers, by occupying a wooden chaise longue on deck. He managed to go below to hold a brief service on Sunday, November 11, his last sermon in the army—"Humility, Not Hubris, in the Post-War World." "A few enlisted men came, no officers. No one listened." Otherwise, life on deck captured all of his attention. He wanted to go home. Yet he had had another "home" since March 1943—the 102nd Evac. And while this movable home had brought him trauma, sorrow, and at least temporary depression, it had also afforded him an invigorating adventure—and that was what he focused on as he sat in that deck chair wrapped in two wool blankets and clutching his diary. At the back of the diary he scribbled notes—one- and two-line vignettes about happy times with the Bull, the Brow, and the Brain. He then rewrote portions of the manuscript, "The History of the 102nd Evacuation Hospital," inserting more of these uplifting moments. He monitored the voyage of the *Sea Porpoise.* November 5: "Rock of Gibraltor [*sic*] in distance . . . sun shining upon it . . . hills of Spain on north, Africa on south." November 6: "Rough, ship rolling, rain . . . sea a slate color but white foam and pale green around the ship . . . watch sea." November 9: "Pass some of the Azores . . . stormy weather and great waves but then sun comes out . . . rainbows beautiful, four at once [and] often one in spray of ship . . . seaweed in water indicates we are [now] in the Gulf Stream." November 12: "Quiet sea, band of moonlight on water." Nevertheless, his eyes were not just on the horizon leading to home. That *ultimately* proven companion in life with the 102nd—"My Watch," the "fine Lathan military wrist watch"—still had his compulsive attention as they plowed through the changing time zones. "November 11: "Turn watch back one hour again tonight; have retarded watch one hour on Sun., Mon., Wed., Thur, and Sat nights—five times." November 12: "Retard again tonight, sixth time." The *Sea Porpoise* had entered the Eastern Standard Time Zone.

Coda

"Home, Again"

Susan and I came home to Birmingham in the late summer of 2008. Two weeks later we drove down to Oak Hill. For some twenty years now my generation of the family has owned the house. It's a special place with over 150 years of family history just as complex as that of the county surrounding it. We could check up on some cousins and perhaps even introduce Pennie of Pennedepie to folks down at the store. It had been a year since I had heard that gentle backhanded humor at the cash register. "I have to say, Tennant, this has to be the first French talking dog ever to come to Wilcox County. Can she do anything else?" And then I would head on up to the house and park myself in the green rocker next to Ren's and ponder the revisions I needed to make in his story. Well, if Pennie's reception at the store went about the way I expected, the succeeding scene up at the house didn't. Barely beyond the lingering effects of jet lag, I just sat there on the front porch, vaguely focused on how changes wrought by war stare you in the face, both in Europe and in Wilcox, and how the return stares vary so greatly. This, in turn, took me to what it was like for Ren to come home, where he was far removed from his other home—the 102nd. It was fittingly complex.

On Tuesday, November 13, at 11:00 PM the 102nd Evacuation Hospital began unloading at Staten Island, New York. By 5:30 AM the next morning they were asleep back in those familiar Camp Kilmer barracks, forty to a room. Six hours later Ren awoke. After a "good steak dinner" in the officers' mess he telephoned Mary, put his footlocker and bedroll on the Trailways to Selma, got a haircut, then spent the rest of the afternoon in the Officers' Club, drinking beer and eating hot dogs and saying goodbye with Joe Rutenberg and Clark Buckley. The conversation was not easy. After a night of "full sleep" in the barracks despite the drunken "noisy bastards" around him, he and Dan Laws ate a farewell breakfast as Dan's detachment-commander duties required his heading south after

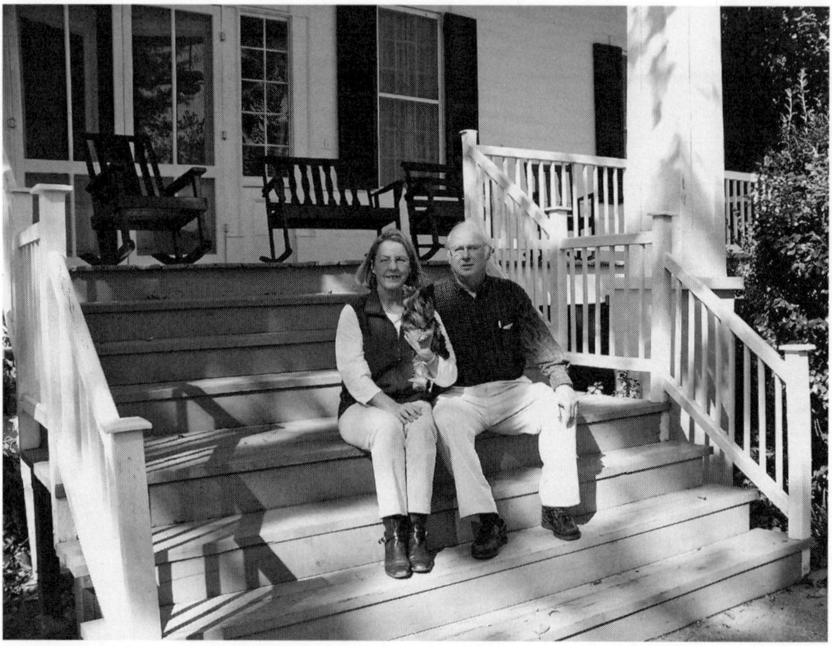

The author, his wife, Susan, and Pennie of Pennedepie at the Jones-McWilliams home in Oak Hill, Alabama. Note Ren's rocker—a double seater—in foreground (November 2010). Photograph by Burk McWilliams.

Ren. That parting was even more difficult. For the next thirty-eight years, annual New Year's Day telephone calls had the Brow and the Pulse still trying to figure out "how we got out of Brest alive" and which one of the physicians "really made the best bug juice." By 4:00 PM Ren and ten others of the 102nd were on a train—the chaplain understatedly designated as "group leader"—for final processing at Fort McPherson in Atlanta. There, as he mustered out, he signed up for the US Army Reserve with a promotion to major, effective October 14, 1946.

At 9:30 AM on Monday, November 19, 1945, Southern Railway no. 37 pulled into Montgomery. Off stepped the khaki-clad minister: fresh haircut, Bronze Star, four battle stars for northern France, the Battle of the Bulge, the Rhineland, and central Germany. Sam's widow, Dot, drove Mary and the girls to meet him. After lunch at The Elite they were back in Camden at 4:30 PM. That night after dinner at the house, where Aunt Joyce and Uncle Bill joined the family, an exhausted Ren managed a few minutes alone in his study. He gave the diary one conflicted distillation: "Home, again." Then early bed.

In some ways it actually was "home, again." Mrs. Tom Moore hosted the Kennedys at "a fine Thanksgiving turkey dinner" with fourteen other guests. The next afternoon old friend Paul Starr came over to join Ren beside the radio for the Alabama–Mississippi State football game, in which Harry Gilmer's leaping passes completed a perfect season and shortly sent the Crimson Tide on to another Rose Bowl victory over Southern Cal. Normalcy in full force. It continued two days later, Sunday, November 25, when Ren returned to his pulpit at the Camden Associate Reformed Presbyterian (ARP) Church. Two hundred fifty people from across the county found seats, and the ushers apologetically turned away more than forty others.

Compared to "The Christian and the War" sermon of 1942 and its theological implications for killing, he was decidedly secular. After emphasizing how important it was for democratic Christians, notably those in the United States, not to make the mistakes in the post–World War II era that had been made after World War I, he explained that his congregations had granted him a "leave of absence" and that "accountability" called for his "report." The sermon ran just over an hour.

He related where he had been for the last two and half years—from Harvard to California to Europe. He explained the differences between army hospitals, evacuation hospitals, and field hospitals. He told of his various roles as a chaplain in war—the preacher in tents and châteaux, the social psychologist and social worker who counseled on divorce, battle trauma, alcoholism, death, and sexual assault. He waxed eloquent on "the sheer amazing experience" of seeing more of "our country" and then "almost all of Europe" alongside "the quick moves, the uncertainty, the excitement, the good companions." He described intense experiences with "heroics . . . the best there is in human nature" and "also the worst . . . suffering, hunger, death, horror . . . details perhaps left [for the time being] unexpressed."

That morning, ten-year-old Betty Gaines sat two rows from the front with her close friends, Lisa McNeill—Sam's niece—and Ren's younger daughter, Margaret. Fifty years later Betty recalled, "The truth is we were at an irreverent age, just little hell-raisers in a small town, with no comprehension of serious matters. But when he got to that part where he said something like, 'The horrible details of death I will spare you,' his voice quivered, and he stared down right at us, and I'm telling you we understood that something serious and horrible had happened." But he didn't stop on that note. With the good and the evil of it all still conflicted within him—which continued the rest of his life—he wrapped up as if the Pulse and the Brow were standing in front of the tents sipping bug juice while probing the modern thought that history happens to everyone and the most balanced, indeed happy people are the ones who consciously make the most of this unavoidable reality. "I don't know what the war has done to me, but I do not regret it." Evac life.

For the next thirty years Ren Kennedy pastored the ARP churches of Camden and Marion Junction and, after 1954, the one at Oak Hill, too. And, following one iconic alteration, this "home, again" seemed to satisfy him. In January of 1947 he took $75 from his US Army Reserve pay, caught a ride with Burford Hollinger to the US Army Surplus Depot near Atlanta, and for the first time bought himself a car—an army Jeep. Ren—behind the wheel of *Alabama III,* smoke pouring out of his Belgian briar pipe, and the most recent "mutt-dog" riding shotgun—quickly became part of the Wilcox scene.

He also stayed devoted to his diary, scholarly reading, and freelance journalism. His writing, of course, included pieces for the *Christian Century,* recollections of Americans in Europe—drunken soldiers killing farm animals just for sport, drunken soldiers wrecking Jeeps and trucks and running over civilians. "Rank . . . and grade . . . make little difference . . . [with] enlisted men making a better showing than officers." Yet the analysis went deeper, reflecting his long-time preoccupation with the "lack of thought" among his 102nd colleagues. Those who "came thousands of miles to fight a bloody war [and] fought it very well" were "great people when there [was] some specific, definite, concrete task to be done." However, they "seldom understood why they were in Europe . . . why [we] fought, nor what victory means . . . and [were] not concerned to understand more." Good and evil seemed of little relevance to most of them. Members of the American Legion nationwide sent letters to Camden accusing him of being "un-American." Quoting him liberally, *Time* magazine praised him for encouraging realistic thought amid the otherwise orgy of self-congratulatory Americanism, which did not bode well for world affairs of the immediate future.

Soon, however, even with liberations afforded by *Alabama III,* he found that he could not be happy doing what he had always done. The enduring impact of life inside and outside the 102nd Evac worked on him. Despite his thoughts on how "unthinking," at times even "odious and disgusting," his GI colleagues had been, the fact remained that he deeply missed them and their surrounding world of war. There was the profound sense of male friendship, which he knew from the extended bug-juice sessions punctuated by that "ack, ack, ack." There was the sweep of history as he walked into rooms where William Shakespeare and, yes, Adolph Hitler had walked. Too, the courage of blown-up Vasco Hale and the brave goodness of Georges and Aimé Talec, Louis Croc, and others of the Ploudaniel Resistance fighters. Equally intense remained his sorrow. Through the deaths of Sam McNeill, Willard Lumpkin, the pilot for whom they needed a bucket, Bleuette Bindell of Sartilly, and others laid out in makeshift graves at Saint James and Limey and still others whose skin wound up on lamp shades at Dachau . . . through these deaths and the multitude of others he felt abject sorrow about the evil that comes from war. Granted, these wretched experiences in which "nothing whatsoever is sacred and anything at all may be violated" ultimately took him "down" below anything he had ever known. But it also was reality. Compared to the way life with the 102nd Evac intensely filled his modern senses, his nonwar life in Wilcox during his first years back left him wanting. At the deepest level, he was having a hard time channeling the impact of history on himself. This worked on him. He understood it, but it worked on him.

To ease these frustrations Ren tried something new. An old friend, Camden native Emmett Kilpatrick, who had been teaching literature at nearby Troy State Teacher's College, was headed for sabbatical. Ren agreed to fill in for him on a part-time basis. In January of 1948 he began commuting several days a week in *Alabama III.* With striking success in the classroom, he started teaching full time in 1953. During the week he lived in an apartment in Troy, ninety miles west of Camden, and handled his ministerial duties on long weekends. He did not want to stop being a minister. He just also wanted to be part of an environment with far more daily talk about great books and compelling ideas, not to mention the freewheeling beer sessions with faculty colleagues about life in general—these things helped satisfy his worldly interests energized by the war. Ren loved Troy and Troy loved him.

So, steadily, time and his happiness over the expanded college life diminished Ren's longings from the 102nd. In 1958 Troy State promoted him to director of public relations and soon after to executive assistant to the president, with lobbying duties in the legislature in Montgomery. In 1961 he quietly emerged as the faculty's choice to become the next president of Troy State. Alabama politics failed to cooperate. Nonetheless, Ren continued to thrive with this intensely secular life during the week and his ministerial endeavors on Fridays, Saturdays, and Sundays. Finally, in 1970, at age seventy and plagued by worsening emphysema, he retired first from academic life and, four years later, from the pulpit. On December 4, 1985, cancer killed him.

During his last two years I visited Ren on three lengthy occasions in his study at the manse in Camden. We agreed that these would be structured interviews about his life. No tape recorder—at least for these—but I could halt him now and then to get my notes clear. He managed me well, just as he had done with more than one *New York Times* reporter. He stayed in blue pinstripe pajamas and had a fading voice, but that accent of Old South and Ivy League still delivered clear thought. The conversations always came back to the moment when he had rolled the dice and volunteered for military service; although the war changed him, he had "no regrets." His 1946 critique of "unthinking" GIs had not changed. He actually quoted the opening lines of a *Christian Century* piece: "He is standing on a street corner in Germany.... He is more than a little pathetic."

However, he was adamant that "there is nothing more important in my life than what I experienced with the 102nd Evacuation Hospital." He went on: "Sure, it made me unsatisfied with life before the war. Before the war I had only read about war. And I had heard big family stories, especially from my grandfather. As a surgeon in the Confederate Army he saw it all. But when I came home, I really *knew about* life and death ... good and evil ... and about war and at least more about issues of moral order and how unresolvable some contradictions can be at a given moment in time." He seemed more focused on his own intellectual development and understanding of humanity through war than on moralistic judgment of others in the context of Christian theology. Toward the end of the last interview he confirmed this: "It still saddens me to know there was something as awful as World War II. But if there was going to be one, I wanted to be there, and I am glad I was. Being with the 102nd was like going to school in reality. I have to say that I may have learned more with the 102nd than I did at Princeton." The chaplain's conflict over the war—how he struggled with its good and evil and related tension between happiness and sadness and logic and emotion—forced this already beautifully educated man to grow into a more worldly and sophisticated human.

With such thoughts it is not surprising that he was intrigued by *M*A*S*H.* I asked him about the character Father Mulcahy. "Not realistic. Too ecumenical. Most of the Catholic chaplains were less interested in being chaplains and more interested in being Catholic and trying to control other chaplains." I asked him about "Hawkeye." "Well, in some ways realistic and in other ways not. Drinking, smart, quick humor, caring a lot about the boys ripped open . . . yes. But most surgeons I knew did not worry about big issues of war. They worried about how much money the war was costing them." I pressed back: "I know of some physicians who weren't like this; they were there because they wanted to be." He retorted, "I said *most* doctors. I'll grant there were exceptions . . . for example, Ed Peterson, and he had medical school debts to pay off, but most were not like Ed." Still, his overarching devotion to the 102nd never went away. Nor—to answer a question I had pondered for a while—did his Christianity. Compulsively organized to within several weeks of his death, he used a notebook to remind him of people dead and still living for whom he wanted to offer birthday prayers. Here with his family and Wilcox comrades I found John F. Kennedy and Paul "Bear" Bryant, alongside 1st Lt. Amy Erickson, Capt. Joe Rutenberg, Pvt. Sam McNeill, Capt. Ed Peterson, Pvt. Roland Rhynus, and Capt. Dan Laws. Patton didn't make the cut.

Commentary on Sources

The Renwick C. Kennedy Papers, covering the years from 1927 to 1980, currently remain in my possession. Of the 5,000 letters in this collection, 436 pertain to the 102nd Evacuation Hospital. Some of the long letters he mailed home from the war were lost, but he typed virtually all of these and returned from overseas with a thick stack of onionskin carbon copies. The diaries consist of thirty notebooks, each approximately five-by-nine inches and running some forty pages; five of these cover Kennedy's experiences with the 102nd. His sermons for the war years and otherwise include handwritten updates on when and where he delivered them. Kennedy correspondence, 102nd photos, and biographical documents can also be found in the Roland Rhynus Papers, in possession of Rolinda Rhynus Luevano, Colton, California; Special Collections and Archives, Henry Luce III Library, Princeton Theological Seminary; Special Collections and Archives, Jean and Alexander Heard Library System, Vanderbilt University; Southern Historical Collection, H. W. Wilson Library, University of North Carolina; Archives and Special Collections, McCain Library, Erskine College and Seminary; Alabama Department of Archives and History; Archives of the US Army Chaplain Center and School, Fort Jackson, Columbia, South Carolina; Sam McNeill Papers, in possession of Fleetwood Hollinger, Camden, Alabama; Russell E. Summerlin Papers, Delta, Alabama (in his possession), and Emmett Kilpatrick Papers (privately held). The Military Records Division of the National Archives, College Park, Maryland, holds the Records of the Office of the Surgeon General, which contain standard periodic reports filed by commanding officers of the 102nd Evacuation Hospital, the 75th Medical Battalion Armored, and the 240th Medical Battalion, as well as Reports of Operations (Medical) for the First, Third, and Ninth US armies. Also at the Military Records Division of the National Archives, College Park, Maryland, is the final version of "The History of the 102nd Evacuation

Hospital (SM)." The authors cited in it are Kennedy, Lt. Betty M. Baker, and Lt. Laverne Clare, but from Kennedy's diaries it appears that he was the chief author from start to finish. Likewise located at this National Archives facility are the Records of the Chief of Chaplains, which include Kennedy's "201" (personnel) file and most of Kennedy's "Monthly [Chaplain] Reports." The horrible fire at the National Personnel Records Center in St. Louis, Missouri, apparently destroyed official rosters and many of the "201 files" of the 102nd, though not that of Carlton D. Goodiel. Three file folders reflecting the daily operations of the 102nd are in the Business Archives of Château de Roumont, Ochamps, Belgium, under the supervision of Jean-Christophe Coppée. The diary of Christine Châteauneuf Croc, which pertains to the 102nd's operations in and around Ploudaniel, France, is in possession of Sylvie Louboutin-Croc, of Ploudaniel, France.

People on both sides of the Atlantic—in most cases people who will never meet each other despite sharing an intense bond—provided interviews key to reconstructing the details and the setting for Captain Kennedy and the 102nd. They are as follows: Mary Conway Kennedy Dickinson of Atmore, Alabama; Margaret Kennedy Ausley of Nokesville, Virginia; Richard N. Kennedy of Atlanta, Georgia; Charles S. Carlisle of Due West, South Carolina; Lowry Ware of Due West, South Carolina; John Brinsfield (historian, Army Chaplain Center and School, Fort Jackson) of Columbia, South Carolina; John Laurie Dale of Oak Hill, Alabama; Betty Gaines Kennedy of Camden, Alabama; Fay Dale Browning of Oak Hill, Alabama, and Washington, DC; Robert and Juliette Harper Bullock of Oak Hill, Alabama; Fleetwood Hollinger of Camden, Alabama; Jane Shelton Dale of Camden, Alabama, and Bonclarken, North Carolina; Lisa McNeill Dobson of Camden, Alabama; Robert Jefferson of Birmingham, Alabama; Margaret Ann Peterson of Birmingham, Alabama; Rolinda Rynus Luevano of Colton, California; Ann Marie Laws Walton of Elizabethton, Tennessee; Brig. Gen. (ret.) Russell E. Summerlin of Delta, Alabama; Matthew Tinker of Southport, England; Louis Forget of Jullouville, France; Sylvie Louboutin-Croc of Ploudaniel, France; the late Georges Talec of Ploudaniel, France; Daniel Berthou of Ploudaniel, France; Jean Touzé of Saint-Pair-sur-Mer, France; Roland Dulins Duprey of Saint-Pair-sur-Mer, France; Marie-Thérèse Provost Desroches of Saint-Pair-sur-Mer, France; Dominique Bindell Lucas of Saint-Martins-des-Champs, France; Yvette Bindel Gilbert of Caen, France; Marie Louise Lévi-Ménard of Bréville-sur-Mer, France; Fred

Fey of Ettelbruck, Luxembourg; Anne Vincott Bellec of Ploudaniel, France; and Margaret Delaney of Crosby, England.

Long before the *M*A*S*H* phenomenon, high-profile popular journalism drew America's attention to the evacuation efforts of World War II. First came Margaret Bourke-White's "Evacuation Hospital," published in *Life* (February 21, 1944), with striking photos of the 38th evac in Italy. Next, just before marrying Ernest Hemingway, Mary Welsh profiled the evac as a key component in the "chain of evacuation" in "Invasion Medicine: General Hawley Provides Quick Care for Wounded," also published in *Life* (June 19, 1944). Then Bourke-White devoted a full chapter to evacs and the 38th in her widely acclaimed memoir, *They Called It "Purple Heart Valley"* (New York: Simon and Schuster, 1944). The story was off and running. Scholarly histories of evacuation hospitals, including their evolution over three centuries to a climactic association with the US Army in the wars of the mid-twentieth century, include Jonathan D. Hood's "Jonathan Letterman and the Development of a Battlefield Evacuation System" (PhD dissertation, Texas Tech University, 2004); Jonathan H. Jaffin's "Medical Support for the American Expeditionary Forces in France during the First World War" (Master's thesis, US Army Command and General Staff College, 1991); Graham A. Cosmos and Albert E. Cowdrey's *The Medical Department: Medical Service in the European Theater of Operations* (Washington, DC: Center of Military History, US Army, 1992); John H. McMinn and Max Levin's *Medical Department: Personnel in World War II* (Washington, DC: USGPO, 1963); Clarence McKitrick Smith's *The Medical Department: Hospitalization and Evacuation, Zone of Interior* (Washington, DC: US Dept. of the Army, Office of the Chief of Military History, 1956); Richard V. N. Ginn's *The History of the U.S. Army Medical Service Corps* (Washington, DC: Office of the Surgeon General and Center of Military History, US Army, 1997); Mary T. Sarnecky's *History of the U.S. Army Nurse Corps* (Philadelphia: University of Pennsylvania Press, 1999); and Judith A. Bellafaire's *The Army Nurse Corps in World War II* (Washington, D.C.: Kessinger, 2004).

The "Lessons Learned" studies sponsored by the US Military Strategic Information Center at Fort Belvoir, Washington, DC, includes strategic analyses of selected evacuation hospitals (excluding the 102nd) of World War II, Korea, and Vietnam. Still, the crucial primary document for the evac is the US Surgeon General's *Medical Field Manual: Mobile Units of the Medical Department* (Washington, DC, 1942), which contains vivid diagrams and other descriptives of evac procedures.

Four relatively recent works begin to get at modern concerns (e.g., gender discrimination, depression) in evac life, although still on a general level: the masterful three-volume *Encyclopedia of the American Military* (New York: Scribner's, 1994), edited by John E. Jessup and Louise Ketz, which also traces the evolution away from the historic evac into the contemporary combat support hospital (CSH) and the "buddy system" used by every soldier trained as a medic; Albert E. Cowdrey's lucidly distilled *Fighting for Life: American Military Medicine in World War II* (New York: Free Press, 1994); Mary Sarnecky's *History of the U.S. Army Nurse Corps* (Philadelphia: University of Pennsylvania Press, 1999); and Judith Bellafaire and Mercedes Herrera Graf's *Women Doctors in War* (College Station: Texas A&M University Press, 2009), which documents no female physicians in evacs until two "slipped through" in Vietnam. On December 2 and 3, 2008, the North Atlantic Treaty Organization sponsored a conference in Siegburg, Germany, titled "Medical Challenges in the Evacuation Chain." Available online, the papers from this conference show how far "evacuation" has evolved since World War II.

Standard recent works on the flow of battles on the western front helped form a framework for the movement of the 102nd evac through France, Belgium, Luxembourg, and Germany. These include Stephen E. Ambrose, *Citizen Soldiers* (New York: Simon and Schuster, 1997) and *D-Day, June 6, 1994* (New York: Simon and Schuster, 1994); John Keegan, *Six Armies in Normandy* (New York: Viking, 1982); and Russell F. Weigley, *Eisenhower's Lieutenants: The Campaign of France and Germany, 1944–1945* (Bloomington: Indiana University Press, 1981). Carlo D'Este's *Eisenhower: A Soldier's Life* (New York: Holt, 2002) assisted in this regard, too. More helpful, however, just for the level of detail, were three volumes in The United States Army in World War II series: Martin Blumenson's *The European Theater of Operations: Breakout and Pursuit* (Washington, DC: Office of the Chief of Military History, Dept. of the Army, 1961); Hugh M. Cole's *The Ardennes: The Battle of the Bulge* (Washington, DC: USGPO, 1965); and Charles B. MacDonald's *The Last Offensive* (Washington, DC: Office of the Chief of Military History, US Army, 1973).

Even greater local detail about the movements of the 102nd came from the works of highly skilled, nonprofessional historians in Europe, such as Jeanne Leboulleux-Léonardi, *Ploudaniel: Une Histoire* (Saint-Thonan: Cloître Imprimeurs, 2005); *Saint-Aubin-des-Préaux: Son Histoire* (Granville: La Fédération de la Manche des Retraités, 1991); Edith Bertin and Jacques Bertin, *Evence Coppée III, 1882–1945* (Brussels, 1991); Fred Fey,

"L'École Agricole de l'État pendant la Deuxième Guerre Mondiale," in *125 Ans: Lycée Technique Agricole d'Ettelbruck,* ed. Lycée Technique Agricole (Luxembourg: Imprimerie Centrale, 2008); and Georges Talec, "La Résistance dans le Secteur de Lesneven," unpublished manuscript (Ploudaniel, 1989).

In addition, there are memoirs, diaries, and collections of letters telling the evac story from the perspective of physicians and nurses. Those of the World War II era that helped the most in this study include Zachary Friedenburg's carefully written *Hospital at War: The 95th Evacuation Hospital in World War II* (College Station: Texas A&M University Press, 2005); Charles Fyfe Stewart's *The Ninth Evac* (New York: Vantage, 1990), LeGette Blythe's *38th Evac* (Charlotte, N.C.: Heritage, 1966); Frank Peyton's *A Surgeon's Diary: 15th Evacuation Hospital* (Lafayette, Ind.: Author, 1987); Max S. Allen and Dan Givan's *Medicine under Canvas: A War Journal of the 77th Evacuation Hospital* (Kansas City, Mo.: Sosland, 1949); Evelyn Monahan and Rosemary Neidel-Greenlee's *And If I Perish: Frontline U.S. Army Nurses in World War II* (New York: Knopf, 2004); and the early one rarely cited today but filled with detail and flair, Clifford L. Graves's *Front Line Surgeons* (San Diego: Frye and Smith, 1950).

In general, these memoirs and others like them are stronger on strengths than on weaknesses of the evacs. On the iconic story of Vasco Hale, see Robert F. Jefferson's *Fighting for Hope: African American Troops and the 93rd Infantry Division in World War II and Postwar America* (Baltimore: Johns Hopkins University Press, 2008). Tom Brokaw's *The Greatest Generation* (New York: Random House, 1998), which is certainly not focused exclusively on evac life, still includes lengthy, vivid descriptions of a surgeon and several nurses.

Robert L. Gushwa's *The Best and Worst of Times: The United States Army Chaplaincy, 1920–1945* (Washington, DC: Office of the Chief of Chaplains, Dept. of the Army, 1977) is a nonanalytical narrative that nevertheless sets the scene for chaplains in evacs. Also useful is Wallace M. Hale's well-written chaplain memoir, *Battle Rattle* (Allen, Tex.: Timberwolf, 2004). On the other hand, the library of the US Army's Chaplain Center and School at Fort Jackson, led by John Brinsfield, includes a beautifully organized and rich array of biographical studies assisting such analysis. Kennedy's own war recollections include, as discussed, "The Conqueror," *Christian Century* 16 (April 17, 1946), 495–97, which was profiled in *Time* 47 (May 6, 1946), 24; as well as "How Good Were the Army Chaplains?" *Christian Century* 63 (June 5, 1946), 716–17; "To the Victor

Go the Spoils," *Christian Century* 63 (July 31, 1946), 936–37; "Brass Hats," *Christian Century* 63 (October 2, 1946), 1179–80; and "Military Training for Your Son?" in *Better Homes and Gardens* 25 (October 1946), 33. Eric Goldman's early scholarly attention to Kennedy's dissent from postwar America's self-aggrandizement is found in *The Crucial Decade—and After, 1945–1960* (New York: Simon and Schuster, 1956), 34.

The town Kennedy left and then came back to after the war, Camden, Alabama, is treated in wide-ranging journalism and scholarship: Some of this provides sensitive and accurate portraits of life there during World War II, whereas some of this material is one dimensional and superficial. The noted Viola Goode Liddell, Kennedy's next-door neighbor, published courageous memoirs of the time. Morton Rubin's *Plantation County* (Chapel Hill: University of North Carolina Press, 1951; rev. ed., 1963), originating as one of the Rosenwald-funded dissertations at the University of North Carolina, focuses on Camden in the late 1940s but includes information on the war years as well. As "a young Jewish graduate student from the Northeast researching race and religion in Wilcox County," Rubin told me, "I was protected and assisted by both Kennedy and your uncle [William J. Jones]." Clinton McCarty's *The Reins of Power* (Tallahassee: Sentry, 1999) focuses on even more recent times but also has a perceptive treatment of Camden during the 1940s.

As for the iconic fictional version of evac life, *M*A*S*H,* most of the writings about this series focus on changing plot lines and the evolving stories of the cast. See, for example, David S. Reiss's *M*A*S*H: The Exclusive Inside Story of TV's Most Popular Show* (New York: Bobbs-Merrill, 1980) and Suzy Kalter's *The Complete Book of M*A*S*H* (New York: Abrams, 1984)—informative and enjoyable books in the context of what they are intended to be. Far more probing is James H. Wittebols's *Watching M*A*S*H, Watching America: A Social History of the 1972–1983 Television Series* (Jefferson, N.C.: McFarland, 2003). By design, however, Wittebols's is more an analysis of changing social values inside American culture during the 1970s and early 1980s than a portrait of war's reality inside an evac.

Index